The Phonetic Transcription of Disordered Speech

Two week loan

Please return on or before the last date stamped below.
Charges are made for late return.

The Phonetic Transcription of Disordered Speech

Martin J. Ball, Ph.D.
University of Ulster

Joan Rahilly, Ph.D.
Queen's University of Belfast

Paul Tench, Ph.D.
University of Wales, College of Cardiff

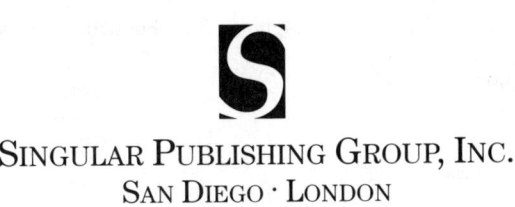

SINGULAR PUBLISHING GROUP, INC.
SAN DIEGO · LONDON

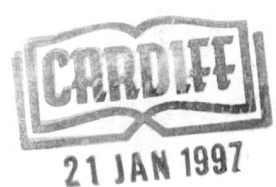

Singular Publishing Group, Inc.
4284 41st Street
San Diego, California 92105-1197

19 Compton Terrace
London, N1 2UN, UK

© 1996 by Singular Publishing Group, Inc.

Typeset in 10/12 Times by So Cal Graphics
Printed in the United States of America by McNaughton & Gunn

Library of Congress Cataloging-in-Publication Data

Ball, Martin J. (Martin John)
    The phonetic transcription of disordered speech / Martin J. Ball,
Joan Rahilly, Paul Tench.
      p. cm.
    Includes bibliographical references and index.
    ISBN 1-56593-206-4
    1. Speech disorders. 2. Phonetics.   I. Rahilly, Joan.
II. Tench, Paul. III. Title.
    [DNLM: 1. Speech Disorders—diagnosis. 2. Phonetics. WM 475
B187p 1995]
RC423.B284   1995
616.85'5—dc20
DNLM/DLC
for Library of Congress
                                      95–31737
                                        CIP

Contents

Preface

This book reflects the increased interest and research into the area of impressionistic transcription of speech and especially the transcription of disordered speech. As we note, there has been considerable development in the provision of symbolization for speech-language pathologists transcribing a wide range of disorders that present in the clinic. However, such provision is wasted, if clinicians do not have access to it and if students are not trained in its use. We, therefore, illustrate the use of phonetic transcription with a wide range of disorders, showing that it is important to transcribe accurately and in detail, to avoid misanalysis and potentially wrong diagnosis. Our aim in this book, then, is to introduce symbol sets for the transcription of disordered speech and voice quality, and set them in the context of the development of phonetic transcription as a whole. We show that transcription is not restricted to the segmental level, but is important at the prosodic level and the discourse level, and we include some advice for teachers as to how they might use available materials to instruct students in the acquisition of transcription skills.

In the first chapter, we look at the history of phonetic transcription, concentrating on the development of the International Phonetic Alphabet (IPA) over the last hundred years or so, the Americanist tradition in transcription, and the various suggestions that have emerged for the transcription of prosodic features of speech. The second chapter explains the central aims, requirements and methods of speech transcription with particular reference to the clinical context. It discusses transcription in relation to phonetics and phonology, and shows how it can inform both, and act as a bridge between these levels of analysis.

Chapter 3 describes a range of methods which might be used to train students in phonetic transcription, and provides details of a range of audio-visual aids and computer-based self-teaching packages that can help with the development of practical phonetic skills.

The following two chapters concentrate on disordered speech and the clinical use of phonetic transcription. In Chapter 4, a range of atypical articulation types is explored, and it is shown how existing and recently developed symbol systems can be used to denote them. Chapter 5 presents a range of clinical data covering many different speech disorders, and shows how the symbols described in previous chapters can be used to transcribe the data. It also stresses the importance of narrow, detailed, transcription, demonstrating how phonemic transcriptions can produce erroneous analyses.

The next three chapters are concerned with transcription above the level of the segment. Chapter 6 deals with a wide variety of symbolizations that have been proposed for the range of prosodic features (including stress, intonation, voice quality, tempo, etc.), while Chapter 7 applies this approach to disorders of prosody, looking in particular at the intonation of the deaf. Chapter 8 extends this account to the level of conversation, looking at ways in which discourse structure can be modeled through transcription: examining both normal and disordered conversation.

The final chapter looks at how transcription and practical phonetics training might develop in the future, in particular through computer-aided analysis. A system is described where acoustic and articulatory information about each phonetic symbol is stored on a microcomputer, and so can be compared to data collected by the transcriber and so aid decisions on which symbol best matches a portion of that data.

This book is aimed at the teacher of courses in practical phonetics, especially those on speech-language pathology programs. However, we hope that it will also be of use to the advanced student, as a way of explaining the importance of accurate and detailed phonetic transcription of clinical data, and as a source book on the latest symbol systems available and ways of learning how to use them. We have continually found that time expended in accurate and detailed description of a speech disorder, whether at segmental or prosodic level, is paid back through accurate diagnosis and therefore more time-effective and appropriate intervention.

CHAPTER

1

The History of Transcription

We talk about everything. When we write, however, we cannot capture on paper everything we say. We cannot capture very easily, for instance, changes in intonation and rhythm, or changes in speed or loudness, or the lowering and raising of the pitch of the voice, or changes in voice quality as we speak.

When we write, we do, of course, record all the words we use, even slang and interjections like *oops* and *aargh*. We record the words in their clauses and sentences and in their paragraphs and whole texts. But we do have difficulty when we want to write about the sounds we use in language. We can easily identify differences in sounds, for instance, at the beginning of the words *this* and *thistle*; and as we talk, we can demonstrate them and contrast them. But it *is* difficult to record these differences on paper without using special symbols. Also, we might wish to draw attention to the similarity between the middle consonant of *measure* in English and the first consonant of *jamais* in French; using a single, universal, symbol for the sound would be very useful.

We are often conscious of differences in accents, too. When we are talking, we can easily imitate the typical British and American variations of words like *class, hot*, and *city*; but if we wanted to write about them, we would be in some difficulty without a knowledge of phonetics and a set of symbols.

Yet another, professional, need for recording the details of speech is when we wish to record deviations of pronunciation in disordered speech. In this realm especially we find it very difficult to cope without special symbols.

1

The use of special symbols for identifying specific details of pronunciation is known as phonetic transcription. If we record the actual words of a stretch of speech, usually from audio recording—whether monologue or dialogue, formal or colloquial, face-to-face or electronically conveyed—that record is usually known as a *transcript*. But if we record the actual details of the pronunciation of those words, that record is usually known as a *transcription*.

We can transcribe a person's pronunciation of single words, and whole sentences. We can transcribe just parts of words, or even just single sounds, or even aspects of single sounds. We can transcribe words in any language or dialect. One very interesting use of transcription is in the preliminary analysis of the sound system of a language that has not yet been reduced to writing. Transcription is a basic procedure in many professional tasks involving a careful analysis of pronunciation: speech therapy, dialect study, forensic analysis of speaker recognition, language learning and teaching, language description, historical linguistics, as well as the ethnographic (or anthropological) study of unwritten languages.

Alphabets

People have always felt—from the earliest human records—there to be an advantage in writing things down. What knowledge we have of our earliest human ancestors is, of course, based on those earliest human records. The earliest written records seem to reflect business transactions; the advantage of a written record is its quasipermanence, as an aid to the memory, in combating dishonesty, and provision of information for third parties. The records, themselves, are pictograms (or pictographs) that strongly resemble the objects of the message, such as the head of an ox. Pictograms eventually get simplified through common usage and the need for rapid recording; the simplified, conventionalized result is known as an ideogram (or ideograph). Ideograms resemble their referents less strongly and are, thus, less iconic than pictograms.

Ideograms are very common in our present-day culture: consider the ideogram of the sun as it appears on weather charts and cameras—also road traffic signs, washing/ironing instructions on clothing labels, dashboard information in cars, for example. Roman numerals are ideograms; one stroke for one, two strokes for two, and so on; the large V represents a hand, thus five; the large X represents, in a convenient, conventional way, two hands, thus 10.

Logograms are symbols designed to represent words, whether they are iconic-like pictograms and ideograms or noniconic—like Arabic numerals. Although the Arabic numeral 1 is iconic, the other numerals have lost their iconicity completely; a few relics do remain, however, such as the three points of 3 and the four points of 4. The simplification and conventionalization of these designs have otherwise completely detached them from their pictographic origins. Chinese writing is largely logographic (but noniconic); basically, it requires as many logograms as a dictionary requires words.

However, in the development of writing in the Middle East, a different principle emerged: the logogram represented not only a referent, but the pronunciation of the referent. Thus, to take wider examples, Oxford could be represented by the logograms of *ox* and *ford*; Washington by a picture of a person washing and the logogram for *ton*; and so on.

This kind of writing is known as rebus writing. It is still common today in children's puzzle books, with a picture representing the pronunciation (or spelling) of a word rather than the word, itself.

The next stage in the development of writing was the total transfer of the significance of the logogram to pronunciation, alone. Thus, the conventionalized ox head came to represent, not the ox, but the pronunciation of the first syllable; in this case [ʔa] from Hebrew *'aleph*. In time, the Greeks simplified the denotation of the symbol yet further, to the single vowel sound represented by the symbol [a]. Thus, symbols came to represent either syllables—in which the writing system, or script, was known as a syllabary—or single sounds, in a writing system known as an alphabet. The term *alphabet* simply refers to the first two letters of the Greek alphabet, *alpha* and *beta*, which were themselves Greek versions of the Hebrew letters *'aleph* and *beth*. In the modern world, a number of syllabaries are in use, such as Japanese Katakana. But alphabets of one kind or another predominate, for example, the Roman alphabet now used for English and many other European languages, Greek, and the Cyrillic for Russian.

The Roman alphabet was adopted from the Greek and adapted to represent Latin. As the need for literacy spread, the Roman alphabet was adapted to handle the pronunciation systems of other languages. Thus the alphabet was extended for Old English with specially designed new letters like æ, as in *æsc* (= "ash"), and ð, a "crossed" *d* used for the *th* in *father*, and with letters borrowed from the runic alphabet.

However, the invention of printing in the fifteenth century imposed a degree of conformity not only on the shape of letters but also on the selection of letters, and some of the Old English extensions to the Roman alphabet were dropped. Furthermore, the alternate shapes of *i/j* and *u/v* were separated as distinct letters, representing distinct vowel and consonant sounds, as in modern English usage.

The spread of printed material began also to impose a degree of conformity in spelling. Whereas writers from different dialect areas spelled according to their accents, a standard spelling began to be established throughout Britain and in other countries where a single language was dominant. In Britain, this process of standardization of spelling culminated in the publication of Samuel Johnson's *Dictionary* in 1755. Although its primary purpose was to record the contemporary meanings of words, one of the unintended effects was its use as a reference work for spelling; people consulted it as an authority on the spelling of words as well as on their meanings.

There was a time when English spelling reflected English pronunciation fairly accurately on a true alphabetic basis, with each separate sound being represented exclusively by a single letter or a pair of letters (e.g., *ch, sh, th, wh, ee, oo*). Thus, the spelling of *time* represented a pronunciation in the fourteenth century rather like *"teamer"* today; here the letter *i* represented an /i/ vowel, and the letter *e* the neutral vowel /ə/.

The simple alphabetic system for English has been thoroughly undermined by a number of factors that have resulted in the serious discrepancy between modern English pronunciation and spelling. No doubt the chief factor has been historical changes in pronunciation. Pronunciation undergoes noticeable change in each succeeding generation. For instance, whereas *ash* and *wash* once rhymed, the vowel in the second word has changed in a way different from the first. In Southern British English, a word like *class* has a vowel that changed its quality to what is typically found in the first syllable of *father*. Thus there are at least the following variations in the pronunciation of the letter *a* today:

ash

wash

father (and class, in Southern British English)

wall, law

hate

to which can be added other possibilities in unstressed syllables, such as:

above

village

and its involvement in other letter combinations, for example:

hair, hare

heart

learn

beat

head

boat

Another factor that has affected the relationships between spelling and pronunciation is borrowing from other languages. English has displayed a great tendency for borrowing words and the original spelling is often retained. Of the hundreds of examples from French, we can identify *naïve* as a case where the letter *a* helps to represent yet another variety of vowel sound.

A third factor has been scholarly intervention. In sixteenth century Britain, there arose a scholarly fashion of adapting contemporary spelling to reflect more closely the classical origins from which certain words came. For instance, an *l* was added to *faute*, which produced the modern spelling *fault*; in which the added *l* eventually got pronounced. On the other hand, a *b* was added to *dette*, which produced the modern spelling *debt*; but the *b* did not get pronounced. Nor did the *p* added in *receipt*, or the *l* in *salmon*, or the *s* in *island*, or the *c* in *scent*, or the *b* in *crumb*, or the *g* in *reign*, and so on. These spellings reflected etymology as well as pronunciation. Such scholarly intervention had a detrimental effect on the alphabetic principle in spelling.

However, a scholarly intervention of a different kind has had a more positive effect. Noah Webster in 1828 published an *American Dictionary of the English Language* in which he incorporated alterations to English spelling that were intended to reduce irregularities and in a small way return to the simple alphabetic system. British spelling has remained conservative by retaining original forms like *centre, colour, programme, catalogue, defence, grey, tyre*, for example, instead of the new spellings *center, color, program, catalog, defense, gray, tire*.

The huge discrepancy between pronunciation and spelling has had at least two popular repercussions. On the one hand, English-speaking people have invented popular spelling forms that are intended to have a visual impact as a strategy to draw attention to the name of a business or product, such as *Nite Klub, Weetabix, Wile U Wate, Q8*. On the other, English language teachers developed a system of symbols to unambiguously represent the actual pronunciation of words for the benefit of learners of the language. This system is what we now know as the The International Phonetic Association (IPA).

The International Phonetic Association

In 1886, a group of French teachers of English met in Paris and formed an association under the title of *The Phonetic Teachers' Association*, with the aim of popularizing phonetic theory and transcription in their profession. Within a year, a number of other well known linguists and phoneticians of other nationalities joined them, and the international dimension to their membership led them to change their name first of all to *L'Association Phonétique des Professeurs de Langues Vivantes* in 1889 and eventually, in 1897, to *L'Association Phonétique Internationale*. Founding members of the IPA included Paul Passy (France), Otto Jespersen (Denmark), J.A. Lundell (Sweden), Wilhelm Viëtor (Germany) and Henry Sweet (Britain). In 1886, Jespersen suggested that the Association should consider establishing a phonetic alphabet that would be applicable to all languages. This, along with the desire to produce appropriate pedagogical materials, became a principal objective of the Association. The first version of the alphabet appeared in 1888 in their journal *ðə fonetik tîtcər*, together with a set of guiding principles. The journal, re-named *Le Maître Phonétique* in 1889, was produced entirely in phonetic transcription until its demise in 1971; thereafter, the Association's journal was radically restyled, with the title *The Journal of the International Phonetic Association* and printed in traditional orthography, but with plentiful sample texts in phonetic transcription.

The IPA Council undertook the task of creating a comprehensive phonetic alphabet with great vigour with new versions appearing in 1900, 1904, 1912, 1921, 1949, and later. One of the principal aims, as stated in the Statutes (IPA, 1949) has been to achieve the scientific and practical representation of languages as yet unwritten or for which there exists only a defective method of representation. To this end, the IPA was involved in the International African Institute's publication of the *Practical Orthography of African Languages* in 1930. (A fuller account of the early development of the IPA can be found in MacMahon, 1986.)

The five guiding principles enunciated in the IPA's *Principles* (1949, 1–2) have been neatly summarized:

1. Wherever possible, differently shaped letters (not just diacritically modified letters) should be used for any two sounds that can distinguish one word from another in a single language.
2. Wherever possible, a single letter should be used for two sounds that are so similar that they never distinguish one word from another in a single language.
3. Wherever possible, only letter shapes that harmonize typographically with the letters of the roman alphabet should be used.
4. Wherever possible, use diacritics only in four circumstances: (i) for suprasegmental phenomena like length, stress, and intonation; (ii) for marking allophonic distinctions; (iii) where one diacritic can make it unnecessary to design a whole set of related new characters (e.g., with the tilde diacritic to indicate nasalized vowels); (iv) to represent minute shades of sound for scientific purposes.
5. Wherever possible, development of the alphabet should be along lines that accord with the phonemic principle and the Cardinal Vowel system. (Pullum & Ladusaw, 1986, p. xx)

These principles led to the publication of a definitive set of symbols in 1949 (see Figure 1–1). The consonants were arranged in a chart that listed the manners of articulation vertically on the left and the points of articulation horizontally across the top. Voiceless and voiced equivalents of sounds shared a column, with the

Consonants	Bilabial.	Labiodental.	Dental and Alveolar.	Retroflex.	Palato-alveolar.	Alveolo-palatal.	Palatal.	Velar.	Uvular.	Pharyngal.	Glottal.
Plosive . . .	p b		t d	ʈ ɖ			c ɟ	k g	q ɢ		ʔ
Nasal . . .	m	ɱ	n	ɳ			ɲ	ŋ	ɴ		
Lateral . . .			l	ɭ			ʎ				
„ fricative .			ɬ ɮ								
Rolled . . .			r						R		
Flapped . .			ɾ	ɽ					R		
Rolled fricative .			ɼ								
Fricative . .	ɸ β	f v	θð|sz|ɹ	ʂ ʐ	ʃ ʒ	ɕ ʑ	ç j	x ɣ	χ ʁ	ħ ʕ	h ɦ
Frictionless Continuants and Semi-vowels . .	w|ɥ	ʋ	ɹ				j (ɥ)	(w) ɰ	ʁ		

Vowels	Rounded						Front Centr. Back				
Close . . .	(y ʉ u)						i y ɨ ʉ ɯ u				
Half-close . .	(ø o)						e ø ɤ o ə				
Half-open . .	(œ ɔ)						ɛ œ ʌ ɔ ɐ ɶ				
Open . . .	(ɒ)						ɑ a ɒ				

Figure 1–1. 1949 IPA Chart. (With acknowledgment to the IPA.)

voiceless one standing to the left; sounds that were deemed to be typically voiced stood in the middle of the column.

The chart represented a view of phonetic theory that highlighted a traditional three-term label for the classification of consonants. Although the chart retained its authority for 40 years, not all phoneticians were happy with all of it. Some people felt that the Association prevaricated on the issue of tongue shape, that whereas *retroflex, palato-alveolar*, and *alveolo-palatal* were designated as points of articulation, they actually represented differences in the shaping of the articulator, the tongue; but another shaping of the tongue, its grooving for /s/, was not indicated at all. Thus the "theory" highlighted some crucial features and ignored the possibility of two distinct dental fricative articulations: a "flat" variant, i.e., [θ/ð] and a grooved variant [s]/[z].

The chart seemed to assume that languages might never distinguish between two types of [j] or [ʀ], and that certain sounds were more common either by being incorporated into the chart or less common by simply being listed as "other letters." Many felt that the chart was thus too Eurocentric.

The vowels were principally represented as the Cardinal Vowel System. The difficulty in devising a system for transcribing vowels is that, whereas it is possible to pinpoint with some accuracy the position of the articulator for consonants, this position is much less certain in the case of vowels. Furthermore, there is almost an infinity of possible permutations of tongue and lip positions. Daniel Jones's solution in the early years of this century was to devise a system of eight "cardinal" vowels of "known formation and acoustic qualities, which serve as a standard of measurement, and by reference to which other vowels can be described" (IPA, 1949, p. 4). The eight cardinal vowels were designated at four degrees of tongue aperture, known as close, half-close, half-open, and open, for both front and back positions of the tongue. Three back vowels—close, half-close, and half-open—involved lip rounding as their most common realizations. A set of secondary vowels had reverse lip shapes, i.e., rounded for unrounded and vice versa, to which were added two close central vowels, one unrounded, the other rounded. They were numbered for ease of reference 1 to 8 for the primary cardinal vowels, 9 to 16 for the equivalent secondary vowels, with the two central vowels numbered 17 and 18. Figures 1–2 and 1–3 show the primary and secondary cardinal vowels.

These symbols were used not only for those precise degrees of aperture but also for tongue positions that are relatively close to them. The IPA sanctioned the use of diacritical marks to indicate more precise positions of the tongue if it was felt necessary:

ẹ for a closer variety (changed in 1989 to e̝)

ę for an opener variety (changed in 1989 to e̞)

ë for a centralized variety

e̽ for a mid centralized variety (introduced in 1989)

e̠ for a retracted variety

o̟ for an advanced variety

and similarly to indicate degrees of lip rounding:

o̹ for a more rounded variety

o̜ for a less rounded, more spread variety

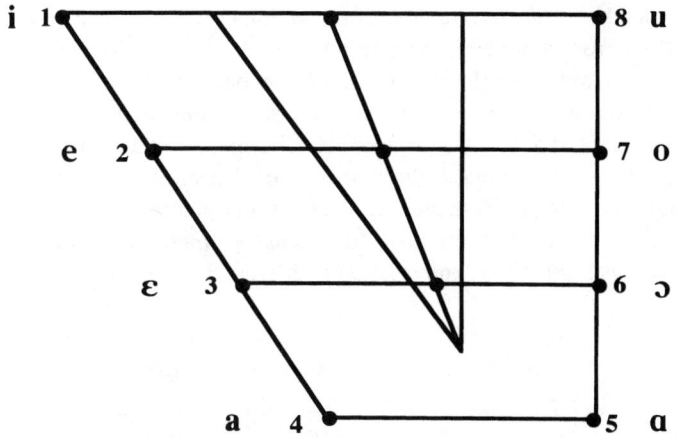

Figure 1-2. Primary Cardinal Vowels.

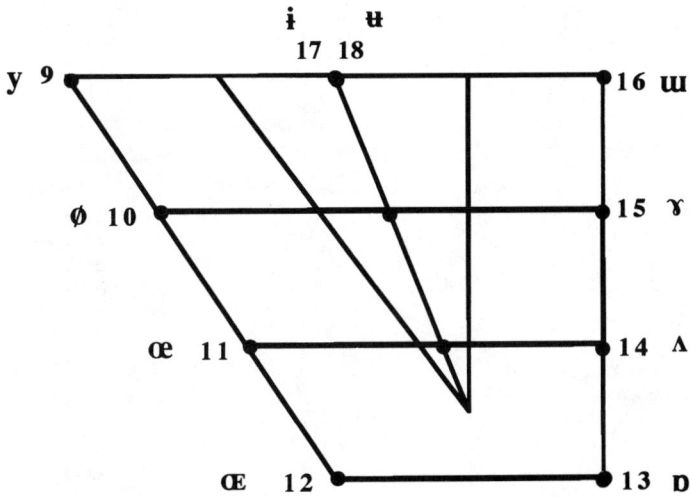

Figure 1-3. Secondary Cardinal Vowels.

One important advantage of the Cardinal Vowel System was that it was not overtly linked to any one language. However, certain other vowel sounds were common in European languages, and special, noncardinal, symbols were sanctioned for the English vowels in *pit, pat, put, a* (unstressed) and the final vowel in *sofa*, for example.

In 1989, a comprehensive review of the alphabet was undertaken to account for observations from a wider range of languages and new insights into phonetic theory and to attempt to settle controversies and perceived contradictions. The resultant, revised, chart of 1993 looks a good deal fuller than that of 1949; the relatively redundant alveopalatal column has disappeared, the central triangle of the vowel chart has been plotted, the non-pulmonic consonants are presented in their own right, and the suprasegmental features and diacritics are arranged systematically. This new chart is the result of intensive, international collaboration. It is reproduced as Figure 1–4, and is also included in the Appendix.

THE INTERNATIONAL PHONETIC ALPHABET (revised to 1993)

CONSONANTS (PULMONIC)

	Bilabial	Labiodental	Dental	Alveolar	Postalveolar	Retroflex	Palatal	Velar	Uvular	Pharyngeal	Glottal
Plosive	p b			t d		ʈ ɖ	c ɟ	k ɡ	q ɢ		ʔ
Nasal	m	ɱ		n		ɳ	ɲ	ŋ	N		
Trill	B			r					R		
Tap or Flap				ɾ		ɽ					
Fricative	ɸ β	f v	θ ð	s z	ʃ ʒ	ʂ ʐ	ç ʝ	x ɣ	χ ʁ	ħ ʕ	h ɦ
Lateral fricative				ɬ ɮ							
Approximant		ʋ		ɹ		ɻ	j	ɰ			
Lateral approximant				l		ɭ	ʎ	L			

Where symbols appear in pairs, the one to the right represents a voiced consonant. Shaded areas denote articulations judged impossible.

CONSONANTS (NON-PULMONIC)

Clicks	Voiced implosives	Ejectives
ʘ Bilabial	ɓ Bilabial	ʼ as in:
ǀ Dental	ɗ Dental/alveolar	pʼ Bilabial
ǃ (Post)alveolar	ʄ Palatal	tʼ Dental/alveolar
ǂ Palatoalveolar	ɠ Velar	kʼ Velar
ǁ Alveolar lateral	ʛ Uvular	sʼ Alveolar fricative

SUPRASEGMENTALS

ˈ Primary stress	ˌfoʊnəˈtɪʃən
ˌ Secondary stress	
ː Long	eː
ˑ Half-long	eˑ
˘ Extra-short	ĕ
. Syllable break	ɹi.ækt
ǀ Minor (foot) group	
‖ Major (intonation) group	
‿ Linking (absence of a break)	

TONES & WORD ACCENTS

LEVEL		CONTOUR	
e̋ or ˥	Extra high	ě or ˇ	Rising
é ˦	High	ê ˆ	Falling
ē ˧	Mid	e᷄ ˀ	High rising
è ˨	Low	e᷅ ˀ	Low rising
ȅ ˩	Extra low	e᷈ ˀ	Rising-falling
↓ Downstep		↗ Global rise	etc.
↑ Upstep		↘ Global fall	

VOWELS

	Front	Central	Back
Close	i y	ɨ ʉ	ɯ u
	ɪ ʏ	ʊ	
Close-mid	e ø	ɘ ɵ	ɤ o
		ə	
Open-mid	ɛ œ	ɜ ɞ	ʌ ɔ
	æ	ɐ	
Open	a ɶ		ɑ ɒ

Where symbols appear in pairs, the one to the right represents a rounded vowel.

DIACRITICS   Diacritics may be placed above a symbol with a descender, e.g. ŋ̊

̥ Voiceless	n̥ d̥	̤ Breathy voiced	b̤ a̤	̪ Dental	t̪ d̪
̬ Voiced	s̬ t̬	̰ Creaky voiced	b̰ a̰	̺ Apical	t̺ d̺
ʰ Aspirated	tʰ dʰ	̼ Linguolabial	t̼ d̼	̻ Laminal	t̻ d̻
̹ More rounded	ɔ̹	ʷ Labialized	tʷ dʷ	̃ Nasalized	ẽ
̜ Less rounded	ɔ̜	ʲ Palatalized	tʲ dʲ	ⁿ Nasal release	dⁿ
̟ Advanced	u̟	ˠ Velarized	tˠ dˠ	ˡ Lateral release	dˡ
̠ Retracted	i̠	ˤ Pharyngealized	tˤ dˤ	̚ No audible release	d̚
̈ Centralized	ë	̴ Velarized or pharyngealized	ɫ		
̽ Mid-centralized	e̽	̝ Raised	e̝ (ɹ̝ = voiced alveolar fricative)		
̩ Syllabic	ɹ̩	̞ Lowered	e̞ (β̞ = voiced bilabial approximant)		
̯ Non-syllabic	e̯	̘ Advanced Tongue Root	e̘		
˞ Rhoticity	ɚ	̙ Retracted Tongue Root	e̙		

OTHER SYMBOLS

ʍ Voiceless labial-velar fricative	ɕ ʑ Alveolo-palatal fricatives
w Voiced labial-velar approximant	ɺ Alveolar lateral flap
ɥ Voiced labial-palatal approximant	ɧ Simultaneous ʃ and x
ʜ Voiceless epiglottal fricative	Affricates and double articulations can be represented by two symbols joined by a tie bar if necessary.
ʢ Voiced epiglottal fricative	
ʡ Epiglottal plosive	k͡p t͡s

Figure 1–4. 1993 IPA Chart. (with acknowledgment to the IPA.)

The American Tradition

There has been a distinctive American tradition of phonetic transcription that has stemmed not from the aspirations of language teachers but from those of anthropologists who were interested in investigating the culture and language of the indigenous American peoples. The most famous of these scholars was Franz Boas, who edited *Handbook of American Indian Languages*, which was published in 1911. This led the committee of the American Anthropological Association to consider recommendations for a transcription system to be used systematically and consistently in the publication of texts and grammars of such languages. This resulted in the publication in 1916 of a report, *Phonetic Transcription of American Indian Languages*, written by P. E. Goddard, Edward Sapir, and A. L. Kroeber as well as by Boas, himself. The transcription system is to be found, for example, in Sapir's famous paper, *Sound Patterns in Language* (1925), and in Bloomfield's 1933 classic *Language*. As more American scholars ventured further, the transcription system was advanced, as displayed in Bloch & Trager's *Outline of Linguistic Analysis* (1942), K. L. Pike's *Phonemics: A Technique for Reducing Languages to Writing* (1947), Hockett's *Manual of Phonology* (1955), and Gleason's *Workbook in Descriptive Linguistics* (1955). For English, the system was adopted by *Webster's Third New International Dictionary* (1961), Kenyon's *American Pronunciation* (1950), and Trager & Smith's *An Outline of English Structure* (1951).

The most comprehensive charts of phonetic symbols were displayed in E. V. Pike's *Dictation Exercises on Phonetics* (1963), Smalley's *Manual of Articulatory Phonetics* (1963), and Trager's *Phonetics: Glossary and Tables* (1964). The charts of the former are reproduced below in Figure 1–5 as typical of these attempts.

The most notable feature that distinguishes the American tradition from the IPA transcription system is the design of the symbols, themselves. The American symbols, apart from a few diacritics, are all typable on an ordinary keyboard. No symbols have been borrowed from another script. Some of the values of symbols betray their English spelling origins, for example, *r* and *y*; *j* was also used by others with its English value; ñ has been borrowed from Spanish. The vowel symbols are basically those of the IPA primary Cardinal Vowel System, except in two very important respects: firstly, the umlaut [¨] is used consistently throughout the chart to indicate reversal of backness; this is clearly borrowed from German, but extended; and secondly, the degrees of tongue height appear to originate from a description of English vowels.

A second feature of the American system is the consistent use of diacritical marks. Modifications to the cardinal points of articulation are consistently indicated by either a subscript arch for a more forward point or a subscript dot for a more backward point. A bar through a stop consonant symbol indicates an equivalent fricative value. An attached comma indicates a corresponding alveo-palatal point. Single diacritics indicate each of the nonpulmonic air mechanisms: glottal-

Manner of Articulation	Air Mechanism	Voicing	Glottal	Uvular	Labiovelar	Back Velar	Velar	Palatal	Retroflexed Alveopalatal	Alveopalatal	Fronted Alveolar	Retroflexed Alveolar	Alveolar	Dental	Interdental	Labiodental	Bilabial
stop		vl.	ʔ		kp	k̇	k	k(		t̢		ṭ	t	t(			p
stop	aspirated	vl.				k̇ʰ	kʰ	kʰ(					tʰ				pʰ
stop	glottalized	vl.				k̇ʔ	kʔ	kʔ(				ṭ(	tʔ				pʔ
stop	implosive	vl.				k̇ᶜ	kᶜ						tᶜ				pᶜ
stop		vd.			gb	ġ·	g	g(		d̢		ḍ	d	d(			b
stop	aspirated	vd.					gʰ						dʰ				bʰ
stop	implosive	vd.					ɠ/g ᶜ						ɗ/d ᶜ				ɓ/b ᶜ
affricate		vl.				kẋ	kx	kx{					ts		tθ	pf	pɸ
affricate	glottalized	vl.				kẋʔ	kxʔ								tθʔ	pfʔ	
affricate		vd.				ġɣ	gɣ	gɣ{					dz		dð	bv	bβ
grooved affricate	aspirated	vl.								tšʰ			tsʰ				
grooved affricate	glottalized	vl.								tšʔ			tsʔ				
grooved affricate		vl.							ṭš	tš			ts				
grooved affricate		vd.								ɉʝ							
grooved affricate		vd.							ḍẓ	dž			dz				
lateral affricate		vl.											tɬ				
lateral affricate	aspirated	vl.											tɬʰ				
lateral affricate	glottalized	vl.											tɬʔ				
lateral affricate		vd.											dl				

vl.	ᵽ	f	θ							x̮	x	x̣				fricative
vl.		fˀ	θˀ								xˀ				glottalized	fricative
vd.	ƀ	v	đ							g̮	g	g̣				fricative
vl.				s̮	s	ṣ	š̮	š	ṣ̌							grooved fricative (or sibilant)
vl.					sˀ			šˀ							glottalized	grooved fricative (or sibilant)
vd.				z̮	z	ẓ	ž̮	ž	ẓ̌							grooved fricative (or sibilant)
vl.					ł											lateral
vl.					łˀ										glottalized	lateral
vd.					l			l̦								lateral
vd.					l̟											fricative lateral
vl.	M				N			Ñ			Ŋ					nasal
vd.	m			n̮	n	ṇ		ñ		ŋ̮	ŋ	ŋ̣				nasal
vl.		f̆			ṟ̌											flap
vd.		v̆			ř	ṛ̌										flap
vd.					l̆											lateral flap
vd.					n̆											nasal flap
vl.	p̃				ṟ̃									R̲			trill
vd.	b̃				r̃									R			trill
vl.	p<			t̮<	t<	ṭ<									click	
vl.					ł<										lateral click	
vd.	b<			d̮<	d<	ḍ<									click	
vd.					l<										lateral click	
vd.	m<			n̮<	n<	ṇ<									nasal click	
vd.					l̨<										nasal lateral click	

Figure 1–5. Pike's **(A)** Contoid Chart and **(B)** Vocoid Chart. (Reprinted with permission of the Summer Institute of Linguistics.) (*continued*)

Voiced vocoids:

Tongue Height	Front		Central		Back	
	Unrounded	Rounded	Unrounded	Rounded	Unrounded	Rounded
high close	i	ü	ɨ	ʉ	ï	u
high open	ɪ	ü̇	ɇ		ï̇	ʊ
mid close	e	ö	ə		ë	o
mid open	ɛ		ʌ			
low close	æ					ɔ
low open	a		ɑ			ɒ

Voiceless vocoids:

Tongue Height	Front		Central		Back	
	Unrounded	Rounded	Unrounded	Rounded	Unrounded	Rounded
high close	I	Ü	ɨ	ʉ	Ï	Ʊ
high open	ɪ	Ü̇			ï̇	U
mid close	E	Ö	ə		Ë	O
mid open	ɛ		ʌ			
low close	Æ					ɔ
low open			A			

B

Figure 1–5. (continued)

ized (or ejective), implosive and clicks. Capitalization indicates voiceless equivalents of typically voiced consonants and vowels. To avoid redundancy, the
superscript wedge indicates alveo-palatal fricatives on the one hand, and flap
articulation on the other (on the assumption that [s] and [z] cannot be flapped),
and the superscript tilde represents the alveopalatal nasal but also trill articulation (on the assumption that whereas [n] can be flapped, it cannot be trilled).

The American transcription tradition has served linguists, anthropologists
and language teachers for a century. Speech pathologists in North America, however, have generally used the IPA.

Iconic Transcriptions

A number of attempts have been made to devise a transcription system that is not based on the Roman alphabet. This is understandable since the shape of the letters is entirely arbitrary. It was thought that by starting from some "prime" shapes, each representing a particular feature of articulation, it would be possible to construct a table of symbols that was both iconic in nature and also logical in embracing all possibilities. Perhaps the most famous attempt was Alexander Melville Bell's *Visible Speech* (1867), though Sweet also constructed a revised and improved version he called Revised Romic (1880-1881) and George Bernard Shaw sought to invent a similarly designed alphabet for English. The shorthand system of Isaac Pitman was based on the same principles.

Alexander Melville Bell aspired to devise a logical, self-interpreting scheme for the notation of all possible sounds that could then be used as the basis of a truly universal writing system for all the languages of the world. He failed to gain the support of the British government, but he and his son, Alexander Graham Bell, who invented the telephone, traveled to America where they used Visible Speech as an aid in teaching those who are deaf to speak. The whole scheme of Visible Speech is set out in Figure 1–6.

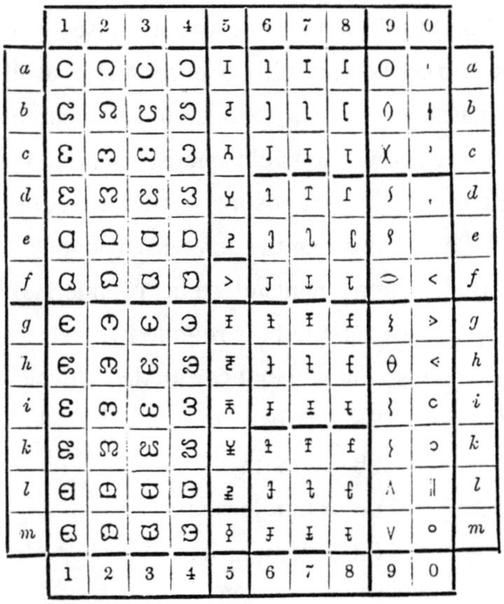

Figure 1–6. Bell's Visible Speech. (From E. J. A. Henderson [1971], *The indispensable foundation*, p. 217. S8, by permission of Oxford University Press.)

The logic and symmetry of the scheme requires a good deal of elucidation. The columns represent, mainly, points of articulation:

1 = velar
2 = palatal
3 = apical
4 = labial
5 = glides
6 = back vowels
7 = central vowels
8 = front vowels
9 = glottal/nasality/modification
0 = prosodic features/air mechanisms/lip shape

The rows represent, mainly, manners of articulation:

a = voiceless fricatives consonants/close tense unrounded vowels
b = voiceless fricative rounded consonants/mid tense unrounded vowels
c = voiceless "divided" consonants/open tense unrounded vowels
d = voiceless "divided" sounded consonants/close lax unrounded vowels
e = voiceless stop consonant/mid lax unrounded vowels
f = voiceless nasal consonants/open lax unrounded vowels
g = voiced fricative consonants/close tense rounded vowels
h = voiced fricative rounded consonants/mid tense rounded vowels
i = voiced "divided" consonants/open tense rounded vowels
k = voiced "divided" consonants/close lax rounded vowels
l = voiced stop consonants/mid lax rounded vowels
m = voiced nasal consonants/open lax rounded vowels

9a = voicelessness   0a = stress
9b = whisper   0b = length
9c = glottal stop   0c = unreleased
9d = nasality   0d = "emphasis"
9e = nasalization
9f = (unclear)   0f = ingressive
9g = trill   0g = ejective

9h = breathy   0h = click
9i = fronted   0i = inverted (lips), i.e. drawn in
9k = backed   0k = protruded (lips)
9l = close   0l = spread (lips)
9m = open   0m = aspiration

Although Bell's Visible Speech is an astonishing achievement, it does leave the modern phonetician puzzled and confused in some respects. For example, "divided" consonants included [l], [s/z] and [θ/ð]. However, the more serious disadvantages include the confusing similarity of letter shapes that the "iconic" principle itself presents and the sheer difficulties of learning the symbols, reading them, and printing them. Certainly, the unfamiliarity of the symbols creates a barrier to the immediate use of them. In any case, as Abercrombie (1967, p. 120) observed, "when such a notation has been learnt, the symbols lose for the practised reader their iconic nature, and function just like any other letters."

The Uses of Transcription

You will have noted that the original stimulus for the IPA was the desire to increase the effectiveness of language teaching and learning, that the original stimulus in the American tradition was the desire to record the languages of North America, and that the ultimate use of Bell's Visible Speech was to improve the speaking ability of those who are deaf. Thus, at least the following uses of phonetic transcription can be identified:

1. Language description and linguistic theory
   (including phonetics and phonology)
2. Language teaching and learning
3. Language pathology

To these we can add:

4. Dialectology and sociolinguistic variation
5. Language acquisition
6. Speech training, elocution and singing
7. Lexicography
8. Spelling reform
9. Reading instruction
10. Literary stylistics

Dialectologists and sociolinguists need phonetic transcription to record variations in pronunciation that are significant in accents, as do psycholinguists to record the development of pronunciation in child language studies. Just as language teachers need transcription to distinguish between conventional spelling and contemporary pronunciation, so do elocutionists and lexicographers. Those who advocate spelling reform base their arguments largely on phonetic criteria, as Noah Webster did. Any theory of reading must, at some point, relate letters to phonetic values; indeed, the *initial teaching alphabet*, a scheme to help young children acquire reading skills, looked very like a transcription. The stylistic potential of sounds as exploited in poetry requires an appreciation of phonetics and reference to symbols.

CHAPTER

②

Transcribing Language

Language transcription is a central tool in speech pathology. As part of the assessment process, speech clinicians must evaluate patients' ability in a range of speech and language tasks: in forming grammatical sentences, in selecting appropriate words for the semantic context, and in producing the sounds that make up a native language, for example. In this book, we focus on the assessment of speech sounds and offer a framework for transcribing speech sounds in the clinical context.

A transcription of speech sounds is valuable to the clinician in 3 main respects: in relation to assessment, to therapy, and in the identification of sound systems that operate in disordered speech. First, the transcription provides a record of patients' pronunciation over a range of speech sounds and it is, therefore, the foundation for clinical assessment of productive ability. Second, it reveals the exact articulatory makeup of the individual sounds or combinations of sounds that are produced. This articulatory information indicates the sounds that are abnormally produced and those that need to be corrected in therapy. It is, consequently, the basis for designing a treatment program. Finally, the transcription offers the potential for revealing important patterns in the data that may be difficult to detect by ear alone. For example, listeners may note that a speaker uses an excessive amount of lip spreading on the alveolar fricative /s/ for example (hence [s̤]) and this may seem to be a random occurrence. Nevertheless, a detailed transcription may well reveal that the labial spreading is common on all alveolar consonants, whether stops or fricatives (hence [d̤] and [n̤], for example).

A transcription, therefore, provides an insight into sound patterns in disordered speech and may indicate a degree of stability in a system that superficially appears to be chaotic. Without a reliable transcription of a patient's speech, a valid assessment or analysis of it cannot be reached, and sensible steps for a remediation plan cannot be taken.

We imagine that most speech pathologists are convinced of the value of transcribing speech for the purposes of assessment, remediation, and identification of systems that we have described above. Nevertheless, they may not be familiar with the various types of transcription that are available and the relative value of each type. This chapter reviews the methods that are available for transcribing speech and explains the contribution of each approach to the assessment of disordered speech. Our central aim is to eliminate potential problems with existing terminology in the field of transcription by offering explanations that are accessible to speech pathology students and teachers. Following these explanations, we discuss the role of phonetic and phonological analyses in assessing disordered speech, highlight the value of an approach that combines both types of analysis, and look briefly at psycholinguistic arguments that underline the importance of looking at phonetics and phonology in equal detail. Finally, we indicate the need to capture elements of social and regional variation in clinical speech analysis and suggest that speech pathology might be valuably informed by elements of sociolinguistic theory in this respect.

Terminology in Speech Transcription and the Need for Clear Explanations

The student who is new to transcribing speech is faced with a range of potentially confusing terms relating to speech sounds and transcription types, such as phoneme, phone, allophone, phonetic, phonemic and phonological. Many textbooks which mention transcription present concise, but rather unhelpful definitions of these terms. Below are two sample explanations of the difference between phonetics and phonology:

> Phonology is the description of the sound system of a language and the link between speech and meaning. Phonetics is the science which studies speech sounds as sounds. Kreidler (1989, p. 13)

> [Phonology is that which] a Frenchman, a Spaniard or an RP speaker acquires in acquiring his native accent, e.g. knowledge about where sounds occur. Carr (1993, p. 13)

These definitions are presented near to the beginning of the texts, at a stage when the learner could be expected to have no prior knowledge of either phonetics or phonology. Although students may be eager to understand the concepts underlying transcription and the concepts of sound organization, they are unlikely to be enlightened when told, rather circuitously, that "Phonetics is the science which studies speech sounds as sounds."

It is likely, therefore, that definitions given early in transcription training, may be of little practical help to students and may even be sources of unnecessary difficulty. Clearly, knowing the definition of any given term is no guarantee of understanding the concept behind it. Grunwell (1987), in a discussion of phonological systems, makes a similar point when she says that "the implications of these terms . . . [i.e. sound patterns in terms of sound elements functioning contrastively] must be properly understood if the concept is to be correctly applied" (p. 86). Above all, teachers should avoid preconditioning students to think that either phonetics or phonology is an inherently difficult subject. Lass (1984), for example, makes the rather daunting comment that "Students often find phonology difficult . . . I'm afraid there's no way out of this" (p. xvii). Although teachers have an obligation to familiarize students with the range of options available for transcribing the speech sounds, we suggest that it is erroneous to get bogged down in theoretical preliminaries and definitions before the central business of transcription begins.

A Method for Training Learners in Phonetic Transcription

A sensible method of training students in phonetic transcription should begin with an immediate emphasis on transcriptional skills in the context of auditory and articulatory training (see Chapter 3 for a detailed discussion of the contribution of auditory and articulatory phonetics to transcription). In a university course, for example, the first 2 or 3 weeks of the semester might be used to familiarize students with techniques of detailed listening, with the symbolization for recording pronunciation and with transcription tasks based on simple aural exercises. It does not matter what label is given to the transcription at this stage, that is, whether phonetic or phonemic, because, in practice, the distinction is likely to make little sense to the learner anyway. In fact, the terms phonetic and phonemic tend to be used rather loosely in many undergraduate courses; what are described as courses in phonetics often do not advance beyond simple phonemic transcription. (The neglect of detailed phonetic training in many institutions is discussed further in Chapter 5.)

Once students are familiar with identifying and transcribing cardinal vowels and consonants, teachers can go on to modify the simple exercises by introducing the idea of variation within individual sound types. This can be done, for example, by presenting words produced in different accent varieties (such as the RP [dʌbᵊldʒɔɪntəd] for *double-jointed*, versus the GenAm pronunciation [dʌbᵊldʒɔɪn̪t̪əd], in which the GenAm /t/ sounds more voiced. Or stretches of speech transcribed in varying detail can be illustrated, as in example 1, taken from Laver (1994, p. 552), in which the term "allophonic" corresponds to the definition of "phonetic" as we have used it thus far.

(1)   Orthographic: These sheep will actually bite the hands that feed them

Phonemic :   /ðiʒ ʃip l akʃlɪ baɪt ðə hanz ðət fid ðm/

Allophonic: [ðiʒ ʃip l̩ akʃlɪ bai̪t̪ ðə hãn̪z̪ ðət fi̪d ðm̩]

Examples such as this demonstrate that, although there are general categories of sound types (identifiable on the basis of their place or manner of articulation), there may be slight modifications in the pronunciation of these types that need to be transcribed to provide a realistic record of the utterance. In the allophonic, or phonetic, transcription in example 1, for instance, the alveolar consonants /t n z d/ are modified in terms of their place of articulation, that is they are dentalized or articulated slightly further forward than the cardinal alveolar position. The vowel /a/, on the other hand, is modified in terms of its manner of articulation; it is not completely oral, but receives a degree of nasalization because of the following nasal consonant.

One may also wish to demonstrate that basic sound types are altered depending on their position in an utterance or depending on the sounds that precede and follow them. Example 2, for instance, illustrates that the general /p/ sound has varying realizations depending on where it occurs in an utterance:

(2)   The pride of spotted lions stunned the Poles

[ðə pʰraɪd əv spɑtd̩ laɪənz stʌnd ðə pʰʷoʊlz]

This example illustrates aspiration of /p/ in initial stressed position, versus nonaspiration in other positions and labialization of /p/ preceding lip-rounded vowels versus nonlabialization in other positions. The realization of /p/ can therefore be shown to be structurally governed by its phonological context, that is its location with respect to other sounds.

Following this method, students' knowledge and experience of transcription will enable them to appreciate the progression from phonemic to phonetic and phonological. We suggest that this progression will provide a more promising basis for understanding phonetic and phonological concepts than will mere definitions.

The approach outlined above whereby students use their experience of one system (phonemic transcription) as the foundation for understanding others (phonetic transcription and phonology) helps them to understand the interrelatedness of concepts in speech transcription, as well as to appreciate the differences between them. This parallels the so-called "network" approach to language teaching and learning described by Ansel and Jucker (1992), as the basis of their HyperLinguistics method. They describe the method in relation to general linguistics learning and define networks as "chunks of information stored in a multitude of interrelations to other chunks of information." The network approach has been shown to be an effective learning technique for general linguistics, and it would seem to offer a valuable method for phonetics as well, if we view phonemic and phonetic transcription and phonology as the particular "chunks of information" that can be networked to give a firm understanding of the concepts underlying the transcription and analysis of speech.

We now move on to present explanations of the central terms in phonetics and phonology. A detailed comprehension of these terms is crucial for adequate transcription, assessment and remediation of disordered speech. In all cases, the explanations are illustrated with examples either from normal or disordered speech.

The Phoneme and Phonemic Analysis

A **phoneme** is a speech sound that is responsible for bringing about a change in meaning. In the Spanish word /pato/ meaning *duck*, for example, there are four separate speech sounds or phonemes, that is /p a t o/. In a second Spanish word /gato/ meaning *cat*, there are also four speech sounds, that is /g a t o/. There are two differences between /pato/ and /gato/: the initial sound in each word and the meaning of the words. When the substitution of one sound for another changes the meaning of the word, we say that those sounds are phonemes. In this case, the substitution of the /g/ sound for the /p/ sound in initial position is responsible for the difference in meaning, so we say that /g/ and /p/ are phonemes and that there is a phonemic distinction between them. A pair of phonemes is also known as a **minimal pair**.

The previous example has illustrated a phonemic distinction in word-initial position, but the distinction can occur in any word position. In Finnish, for example, there is a word-medial phonemic distinction between /kadot/ meaning *failure*, and /katot/ meaning *roofs*. We can therefore identify /d/ and /t/ as separate phonemes, with the voicing contrast between them being responsible for the phonemic difference. In word-final position, a phonemic distinction occurs between the English words /sɪt/ and /sɪp/, for example. Of course, we can also identify phonemic contrasts on the basis of units somewhat smaller than the traditional segment. In Hindi, for example, the feature aspiration is responsible for the phonemic difference between [kʰəl], meaning *wicked person*, and [kəl], meaning either *yesterday* or *tomorrow*. The concept of sound change resulting in meaning change or contrastivity is therefore central to the definition of phoneme.

If the substitution of one sound for another does *not* change the meaning of the word, then the sounds in question are not phonemes so there is no phonemic difference between them and they do not constitute a minimal pair. In a London

Cockney pronunciation of *bottle*, for example, alternative realizations of the word-medial consonant /t/ are [t] and [ʔ], but the substitution of one sound for the other does not bring about a change in meaning. To take another Finnish example, the words /kuzi/ and /kusi/ are differentiated by the third sound, that is the /z/ versus the /s/. Nevertheless, there is no difference in meaning between the words (both mean *six*), so /z/ and /s/ are not separate phonemes in this case and the difference in voicing is not phonemic. When we have two alternative sounds or alternative realizations of the same sound that do not result in a change of meaning, those sounds are in **free variation**.

Phoneticians and speech clinicians are interested in establishing phoneme inventories for any given speaker, because the inventory reveals whether speakers are capable of producing the full range of phonemes that will enable them to make all the necessary contrasts in a language. There are two main factors that should guide identification of a phoneme inventory, whether in normal or disordered speech. Firstly, whether a phonemic contrast exists or not can only be decided on the basis of two different sounds occurring in the same word position (i.e., in **parallel distribution**). Secondly, differences can only be identified based on a single sound difference between two words. One could not, for example, have two words differing in more than one sound and state that it is one particular sound that is responsible for the meaning difference. In Mokilese (a language spoken in Micronesia), for example, [pu̯ko] means *basket* and [poki] means *to strike something*. We cannot state that the distinctions between [u̯] and [o] or between [o] and [i] are phonemic, because the contrast is not limited to one element in the word. In summary, potential phonemes must occur in the same word position and they must be the sole basis for the meaning difference between words.

So far, we have looked at consonant phonemes. But, it is, of course, also possible to identify vowel phonemes. For example, [e] and [i] constitute a minimal pair in Belfast English; the substitution of [e] for [i] changes the meaning from *meet* or *meat* ([mit]) to *mate* ([met]). Vowel length alone may also be responsible for a phonemic distinction. This is the case in Scots English, for example, in which vowel length differentiates *heed* [hid] from *he'd* [hiːd] and *road* [rod] from *rowed* [roːd], for instance.

Normal adult speakers of English possess a phonemic system containing around 40 phonemes (this is the estimate given by Grunwell, 1987, p. 46), that is 40 sounds capable of functioning contrastively. This figure does, of course, vary from language to language (for a discussion of the phonemic inventories in a range of languages, see Laver, 1994, p. 573) and for varieties of English. Nevertheless, 40 seems to be a reasonable estimate for most accents of English, with 24 of these being consonant phonemes. The consonant phonemes are given in Figure 2–1. They are presented from left to right, corresponding to consonant place of articulation from bilablial to glottal:

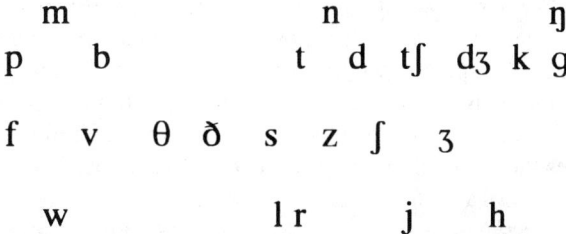

Figure 2-1. Inventory of consonant phonemes.

In establishing the vowel phonemes in English, the situation is more complex, given the wide variety in vowel pronunciation for different varieties. J. Wells (1990) presents vowel phonemes for GenAm and RP and in terms of short vowels, and long vowels and diphthongs. He further identifies six subsections into which these vowels may be divided:

A: / ɪ e æ ɒ ʌ ʊ /

B: / iː eɪ aɪ ɔɪ /

C1: (RP) / uː əʊ aʊ ɒʊ /

C2: (GenAm) / uː oʊ aʊ /

D1: (RP) / ɪə eə aː ɔː ʊə ɜː /

D2: (GenAm) / ɑː ɒː ɔː oː ɜʲ /

Among normal adult speakers, the phonemic system is stable, there is a consistent relationship between sound and meaning. Stability in the phonemic system is crucial for conveying meaning and intelligibility and if the system is impaired, then it is likely to interfere with communication. The instability takes two main forms: sounds may be randomly distributed, with little or no evidence of systematic patterns and may have no apparent relationship to meaning. Example 3, for instance, (from Grunwell, 1987, p. 261) illustrates such a random distribution of sounds in a selection of words produced by a single patient:

(3) finger ['wɪwɪ]

sleeping [wi]

feather ['dɛdɛ]

scissors ['dɪdə]

On the other hand, sounds may be distributed abnormally compared with normal speech, yet they may well follow particular patterns or a system of their own. For example, a speaker who pronounces *north* and *norse* in the same way ([nɔːrs]) and *mouth* and *mouse* in the same way ([maʊs]), fails to make the normal phonemic distinction between [θ] and [s]. Nevertheless if the speaker *consistently* collapses the distinction into a single /s/, the collapse is systematic in itself and therefore follows a particular predictable pattern.

Using the *north/norse, mouth/mouse* examples above, it may be tempting to conclude that predictability and systematicity in a disordered speech sample constitute a degree of normality. It would, however, be wrong to equate systematicity with normality in speech. Although we are likely to know from the context or, perhaps, by familiarity with the speaker which word is intended, irrespective of the realization, it still must be recognized that the speaker's phonemic system has broken down, whether or not that breakdown has a severe effect on intelligibility.

To summarize this section on the phoneme and phonemic systems, we have presented some guidance for identifying phonemes and we have suggested that a stable phonemic system is necessary for normal communication. As we have shown in this section, an analysis and description of any given phonemic system allows the identification of the contrastive sounds of that system. Nevertheless, a phonemic analysis does not allow recording of subtleties of pronunciation that are not responsible for meaning differences. We may wish, for example, to indicate details of pronunciation in speakers from two different geographical regions, in the formal and informal speech of a single speaker, or fine differences in pronunciation in abnormal versus normal speech. To capture such fine differences, phonetic transcription and analysis are needed. This is discussed next.

Phonetics

Phonetics is the study of speech sounds. It is common practice to divide phonetic study into three subfields: auditory phonetics, articulatory phonetics, and acoustic phonetics. Auditory phonetics deals with the perception of speech sounds. Training in auditory phonetics is essentially ear training and practice in auditory phonetics allows us to recognize speech sounds and differentiate them one from another. Articulatory phonetics deals with the production of speech sounds. A knowledge of articulatory phonetics allows us to identify the exact articulatory characteristics of the sounds heard, and allows classification of them into particular categories according to their phonation type and their place and manner of articulation. Acoustic phonetics deals with the instrumental measurement of the physical properties of speech, such as intensity, duration, and frequency. Auditory and articulatory phonetics differ from acoustic phonetics insofar as they provide impressionistic evaluations of speech, whereas the latter provides objective measurement of physical phenomena. The implication of this difference is that listeners may disagree somewhat in their identification of phonetic categories using auditory and articulatory information (variability among phonetic transcribers is discussed in Chapters 3 and 9), whereas acoustic measurements, properly carried out, offer little room for dispute.

Phonetic transcription is the task of using written symbols to reflect the sounds of speech. It is important to distinguish a phonetic transcription from a phonemic transcription. A phonemic transcription is "broad," insofar as it aims to capture broad phonemic contrasts that are responsible for conveying meaning. A phonetic transcription, on the other hand, is "narrow," as it captures fine details in the pronunciation of any given sound (the terms "broad" and "narrow" are discussed in more detail in Chapter 5). A sound may, for example, be pronounced slightly differently depending on the speaker's accent or the stylistic context of the speech event. A phonetic transcription is also known as an allophonic transcription, and whereas a phonemic transcription presents a series of phonemes, a phonetic transcription presents a series of **allophones, allophonic variants**, or **phones**. These terms refer to symbols that capture the exact articulatory characteristics of a sound. To produce a reliable phonetic transcription, listeners require well-developed skills in auditory and articulatory phonetics (methods of acquiring these skills are suggested in Chapter 3).

It will be clear from many of the examples in this chapter that a true phonetic transcription requires more than just the basic symbols for consonants and vowels. If accurate reflection of variation in speech sounds is desired, reference to diacritics is needed. A diacritic is a symbol that indicates some variation in the realization of a phoneme. A centralized pronunciation of a vowel, for example, is indicated by the diacritic placed above the vowel, as in [ä], for example. The segmental diacritics that are sanctioned by the IPA are reproduced in Figure 2–2, with Figure 2–3 showing the location of the diacritically modified vowels on the vowel chart.

In the course of phonetic transcription, one may encounter sounds that correspond to the general phoneme type and have no particular phonetic modification associated with them. For example, the velar plosive /k/ may be realized without any particular modifications to the basic consonant type, as in /kɑɹ/ for *car*, for example and in this case the /k/ phoneme is the correct transcription. In practice, a phonetic transcription will record phonemic and allophonic variation. A phonetic transcription differs from a phonemic transcription, because the phonetic version pays needed attention to the possibility of allophones and notes them if necessary. A phonemic transcription, on the other hand, excludes the possibility of allophonic variation.

In the explanation above, we have used the term "phonetic contrast" to refer to minor changes in place of articulation, such as from alveolar to dental, for example. Of course, it is also possible to identify phonetic differences between

DIACRITICS Diacritics may be placed above a symbol with a descender, e.g. ŋ̊

̥	Voiceless	n̥ d̥	̈	Breathy voiced	b̤ a̤	̪	Dental t̪ d̪
̬	Voiced	s̬ t̬	̰	Creaky voiced	b̰ a̰	̺	Apical t̺ d̺
ʰ	Aspirated	tʰ dʰ	̼	Linguolabial	t̼ d̼	̻	Laminal t̻ d̻
̹	More rounded	ɔ̹	ʷ	Labialized	tʷ dʷ	̃	Nasalized ẽ
̜	Less rounded	ɔ̜	ʲ	Palatalized	tʲ dʲ	ⁿ	Nasal release dⁿ
̟	Advanced	u̟	ˠ	Velarized	tˠ dˠ	ˡ	Lateral release dˡ
̠	Retracted	i̠	ˤ	Pharyngealized	tˤ dˤ	̚	No audible release d̚
̈	Centralized	ë	̴	Velarized or pharyngealized	ɫ		
̽	Mid-centralized	e̽	̝	Raised	e̝ (ɹ̝ = voiced alveolar fricative)		
̩	Syllabic	l̩	̞	Lowered	e̞ (β̞ = voiced bilabial approximant)		
̯	Non-syllabic	e̯	̘	Advanced Tongue Root	e̘		
˞	Rhoticity	ɚ˞	̙	Retracted Tongue Root	e̙		

Figure 2–2. Segmental diacritics sanctioned by the IPA (with Acknowledgments to the IPA).

sounds that are relatively far apart in terms of place of articulation, such as /g/ and /t/ for example. Generally, however, we tend to reserve phonetic contrast for talking about minor differences between sounds.

In disordered speech, one can identify a range of so-called "phonetic problems." Phonetic errors can be classified as a reduction in the range of phonetic contrasts, as distortion of the basic target sound type or insertion of sounds from outside the target language. A reduction in the range of phonetic contrasts is illustrated by Grunwell (1987, p. 260) by way of an 8-year-old child's pronunciation of *digging* as ['tɪtɪn], where the child loses the phonetic contrast between [d] and [g]. Distortion of the basic sound type can be illustrated by way of excessive force in articulation, for example (discussed further in Chapter 7). With regard to

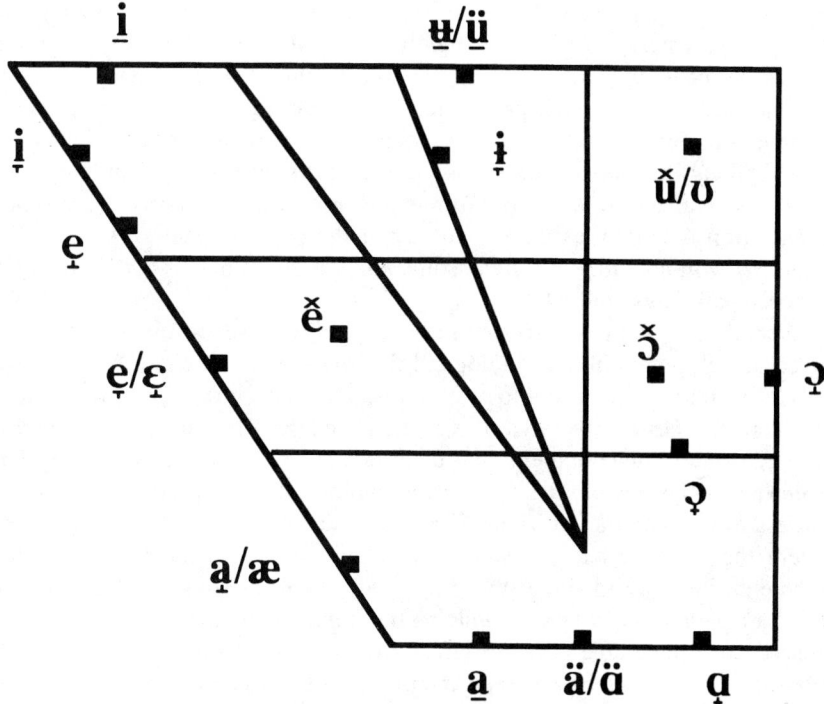

Figure 2–3. Diacritic usage with vowels.

sounds lying outside the system of an individual's native language, one might envisage dentolabial articulations, in which the lower teeth articulate with the upper lip, and bidental articulations, in which the lower and upper teeth articulate together (symbolizations for these and other disordered articulations are given in Chapter 5).

In clinical speech analysis, only phonetic transcription has any validity for the assessment of speech disorders, as it is the only system allowing recording of fine degrees of variation in the realization of any given sound type.

Phonology

The phonemic and phonetic systems of a language operate at a micro level, at the level of individual sounds or features of sounds. We describe a phonemic contrast, for example, as one sound contrasting with another sound by meaning and a phonetic contrast as two sounds being different in their articulatory makeup, irrespective of meaning. There is also, however, a higher level, or macro-organization that operates in speech production and one must be able to record this in transcription. This higher level organization deals with how the realization of one sound affects the realization of preceding and subsequent sounds and how sounds are realized depending on their position in the utterance. This type of organization is known as the phonology or the phonological system of a language. We will now look briefly at some phonological concepts commonly used in speech pathology studies.

Speech pathologists carry out phonological analyses to investigate phonological development and phonological disorders. Phonological concepts were introduced into speech pathology literature and speech therapy training in the late 1960s and Grunwell (1985, p. 165) has stated that the concepts of phonological organization, development, and disorders have become fully established in speech pathology and clinical practice. Phonological analysis attempts to provide answers to two central questions. First, do patients possess a normal phonemic system, that is, is there a consistent relationship between meaning and sounds or is there an inability to signal meaning contrasts all or some of the time? Secondly, are patients capable of producing the full range of phonetic contrasts characteristic of a language? Phonological analysis, therefore, involves a detailed investigation of both the phonemic and the phonetic systems of patients.

Most phonological assessment procedures currently in clinical use are based on phonological process analysis (see the procedures by Grunwell, 1985; Hodson, 1980; Ingram, 1981; Shriberg & Kwiatowski, 1980; Weiner, 1979). Process analysis tells us how the actual pronunciation of the speaker relates to the target sound. For example, the production of a target /g/ as /d/ illustrates a "fronting" of the velar consonant to an alveolar position. Phonological processes fall into two main categories, substitutions (as in the example above) and omissions (with one sound left out, as in [kul] for *school*, [skuːl]).

From what we have said above, it should be clear that the term phonology can be used in two senses. In the first sense, it refers to the effect that phonetic context has on the realization of sounds. In this sense, one can see that phonology and phonetics operate on separate but interconnecting levels and can use our knowledge about the characteristics of connected speech to aid transcription and understanding of the phonetic structure of speech. In the second sense, phonology is an inventory of phonemic and phonetic resources of the speaker. It is clear that both senses of the term involve an explicit relationship with phonetic detail, insofar as both kinds of phonological description call for a detailed phonetic transcription of a speech sample. In the next section, we explore the relationship between phonetics and phonology in more detail.

The Relationship Between Phonetics and Phonology

We have just said that it is possible to differentiate between phonetics and phonology, but that knowledge from phonetics contributes to phonological analysis and vice versa. Although most writers and investigators now agree that phonetics and phonology should be treated as complementary disciplines, this was not always the case. In the past, phonetic study was pursued without regard to phonological factors, and phonologists usually stated that phonetic substance was unrelated to phonological form (for a detailed discussion of the history of phonetic and phonological studies, see Blumstein 1991, pp. 108–119; Diehl, 1991, pp. 120–134). Nevertheless, the 1970s saw an upsurge of phonetically oriented approaches to phonology, with the increasing realization that the study of the sound structure of language would be enhanced by a greater interaction between the study of phonetics and phonology (Blumstein, 1991, p. 110). Along similar lines, Bailey (1985) advocates a field of study called phonetology, which he defines as "a framework in which it is held that neither phonetics nor phonology can be validly carried on in isolation from each other" (p. 141). With particular relevance to clinical speech analysis, the need to investigate phonology and phonetics in equal depth is underlined by Grunwell (1987). She says that "what is required is detailed and compatible phonetic and phonological analyses which must be sensitively interpreted . . . . In this way, information which is more directly applicable in clinical practice will be gained by employing the concepts of phonetics and phonology" (p. 169).

Transcription: The Central Interface Between Phonetics and Phonology

We have suggested above that phonetics and phonology are complementary disciplines and we have summarized the arguments of investigators who argue that both phonetic and phonological analyses should be carried out to arrive at a comprehensive analysis of a speech sample. We now suggest that the major interface between phonetics and phonology is to be found in transcription. We cannot, for instance, arrive at valid phonological assessments (in both of the senses described above) without a detailed phonetic transcription: An inaccurate transcription will have damaging effects on phonological theory (this point is discussed by Bailey, 1978). Bailey (1985, p. ix) also points out that, although many areas of phonetic research have been making great strides forward, phonetic transcription methods have been "moving backwards" and that this has an effect on phonology. Clearly accurate phonetic transcription has a crucial role in phonological theory. In summary, Buckingham and Yule (1987, p. 123), for example, state that, "without good phonetics [by which is meant good phonetic transcription], there can be no good phonology."

The goal of phonemic transcriptions is to identify sounds in terms of linguistic contrastivity. It was this linguistic contrastivity that earlier phonological studies attempted to uncover. Now, however, phonology attempts to deal with contrastivity on other levels, such as social class, regional background, and style. To accomplish this, phonemic transcriptions are inadequate and phonetic transcriptions are called for. The need to use a transcription which reveals contrastivity on a number of other than purely linguistic levels has an added urgency in today's clinical context, in which clinicians are called to judge patients' skills in a range of communicative contexts.

It is, of course, possible to pursue phonetic and phonological transcription and analysis separately from one another. Ryalls, Bédard, Chamberland and Larouche (1993), for example, in their analysis of the speech of a French-speaking child with profound hearing impairment, use only phonemic transcription, because, they state, errors were sufficiently broad to be captured by phonemic transcription. It is also possible to carry out a basic phonological investigation using only phonemic analysis as input, as long as the patient presents with no phonetic errors. A phonetic transcription might be attempted without knowledge of the phonology of connected speech. Nevertheless, one must be aware that one type of analysis without reference to the other is likely to be rather limited. This can, for example, identify patterns that do not adequately characterize a speaker's total system. If one chooses to perform merely phonemic transcription, then one is making the assumption that phonetic errors will not occur, without taking the trouble to verify the assumption. In an attempt to counteract such assumptions, Grunwell (1987) points out that the clinician should be aware that patients might have a phonetic and/or phonological dimension to their speech problems and underlines the importance of using a detailed phonetic analysis on which to base the phonological assessment. She goes on (p. 34ff) to offer some guidelines for the assessment of disordered speech which we summarize here:

Clinicans should:

- Use a descriptive framework/assessment procedure that contains both phonetic and phonological analyses;
- Use a descriptive framework/assessment procedure that will exhaustively analyze the data;
- Record the sample of speech in as detailed a phonetic transcription as possible.

These guidelines further underline the importance of a detailed phonetic transcription in clinical assessment.

Producing and Perceiving Language: The Place of Phonetics and Phonology

The phonetics/phonology division in the assessment of disordered speech is useful in a number of respects. First, the division offers a convenient means of distinguishing between the two main trends in assessing disordered speech, that is transcription and analysis. Clearly, phonetics corresponds to transcription, in which as many details about the production of the speech sounds as possible are captured. Phonology, on the other hand, corresponds to analysis and identification of systems, in which one identifies patterns of pronunciation or sound organization in the speaker's output. The phonetics and phonology division, therefore, provides a comprehensive means of categorizing the two main aspects of spoken language. In this sense, the division is, using Hewlett's (1985) term, "data-oriented."

The phonetics/phonology division is, however, also useful in a second sense. As well as providing insights into the data, it may also contribute to our understanding of the processes that are involved in speech production. In this sense, the division is relevant psycholinguistically, and may be referred to as "speaker-oriented" (Hewlett, 1985). The central question is: How do speakers store sounds mentally? Are sounds stored as general sound types (phonemes) or are they stored as allophones?

Most conventional models of speech production suggest that speakers' mental representation of utterances consists of sequences of abstract descriptions or mental images of sounds. These models suggest that speech is stored as a sequence of separable discrete phonemes. The descriptions or images are transmitted to the vocal apparatus in sequence and each unit sets in motion a set of articulatory motions in the vocal tract. For example, if the sound /d/ is transmitted, then neural impulses control movements in a number of groups of nerves and muscles: closure of the tongue against the alveolar ridge with one group, closure of the nasal passage with another group, and vibration of the vocal cords with another. These models of speech production suggest that language processing operates at the phonological level and that low-level phonetic differences in sound are not encoded in the processing system.

As well as offering explanations as to how speakers produce language, models of speech production also attempt to explain how listeners process sounds, whether it is on a phonetic or a phonological level. Again, conventional models suggest that the phonological level is uppermost, and that listeners process speech on a phonological level by matching sound types with meaning, without regard to the detailed phonetic makeup of the sounds. Given this view of language processing, the basic requirement is intelligibility, that listeners seek to make linguistic sense out of what is said. If the phonological processing breaks down so that the speaker cannot match sound with meaning, communication difficulties result.

The models of language production and processing which rely on phonological explanations are somewhat unconvincing. One of the least satisfactory elements is that they dispense with much of what would intuitively seem to be important for perception and production. Although this book does not seek to offer a detailed psycholinguistic explanation of speech production and perception, we hope to provide a compelling argument for encouraging learners to be concerned with the phonetic level of speech production. In this respect, we suggest that speech production and perception should be concerned with considerably more than issues of mere intelligibility. In speaking and listening to speech, individuals are aware of, for example, the speaker's regional and social background and degrees of abnormality, if presented with disordered speech. It is, therefore, attractive to speculate that speakers and listeners operate on a phonetic as well as a phonological, rather than only a phonological basis.

Our view of speech production and perception as operating on a phonetic and phonological level is supported by physiological studies of speech production. In contrast to the phonological models outlined, the physiological studies suggest that the sequential control of muscles which operate in each sound would be physically impossible if the sounds were produced in a strict sequence (see, for example, Lenneberg, 1967). They suggest that sounds that may appear to be independently produced may, in fact, overlap and may be produced simultaneously. This certainly makes intuitive sense and, in addition, it fits with theories of so-called "parametric phonetics," in which one segment affects preceding and following segments (see Ball, 1993; Laver, 1994).

To summarize this section, we have highlighted the need for detailed phonetic transcription as an important tool in clinical assessment. We have shown that phonetic analysis provides insight into phonological structure and that it is likely to be psycholinguistically relevant on a production and perceptual level.

Providing Adequate Data
for Clinical Transcription

So far in this chapter, we have made the assumption that the speech samples subjected to transcription will be representative of the patients' productive abilities. By "representative" we mean that the samples are wide ranging enough to reflect variability in speech production over a range of speech tasks and a variety of styles, giving a true picture of the speech type in question. Some past studies have suffered from poor data, or poor transcription, or both and the type of data that has traditionally been used in speech pathology studies has tended to be rather formal, often in the form of word lists. However, there is some evidence to suggest that data taken from formal speech is less likely to uncover representative speech disorders than spontaneous speech (Cowie & Douglas-Cowie, 1983; Nilsonne et al., 1988; Douglas-Cowie & Cowie, 1989; Wells, W., 1994). In the case of subjects who have become deaf, Waters (1986) says that it is in informal conversation that the intelligibility begins to suffer. It is therefore possible that the reading exercises and word lists on which most existing studies are based will fail to identify abnormalities that may well occur in less formal language contexts. In the case of verbal dyspraxia in children, for example, Stackhouse and Snowling (1992) found that there was a significantly higher number of segmental errors in connected speech than in single word naming or imitation tasks. According to Brewster, (1989, p. 173), "we need to collect a range of samples from a patient's speech, along a continuum of spontaneous, 'natural' conversation to carefully composed and directed test frames." In particular, speech pathology is increasingly recognizing that it has important lessons to learn from other linguistic disciplines about data selection. Ball (1992), for example, provides a detailed discussion of the relationship between sociolinguistics and clinical speech analysis.

Although sociolinguistic methodology, in particular, offers an important contribution to clinical speech assessment, we also wish to suggest that the detailed phonetic transcription that is central to assessment has a crucial role in sociolinguistics. In contrast to clinical studies, where investigators are increasingly calling for detailed transcription, sociolinguistics tends to present rather superficial transcriptions of pronunciation. Typical analyses refer to phenomena such as /h/ dropping, presence or absence of postvocalic /r/ and the /ɪn/ versus /ɪŋ/ variants (see, for example, Trudgill, 1983, p. 47). Some comments can be even more impressionistic, without reference to any transcription. Holmes (1992, p. 134), for example, says that "the pronunciation of *bath* with the same vowel as in *sat* distinguishes a speaker from the north of England from a southerner." Clearly, the purpose of these sociolinguistic studies is to illustrate very broad differences in pronunciation because of social variables. Nevertheless, we argue that a more detailed analysis of the pronunciation system, especially with respect to vowels, provides a greater insight into the effect of social variation on speech. As was mentioned in the context of disordered speech, a phonemic analysis runs the risk of failing to uncover subtleties of pronunciation that may be relevant for finegrained sociolinguistic distinctions.

This chapter has explained the central aims, requirements, and methods of speech transcription with emphasis on the clinical context. Chapter 3 describes a range of methods that can be used to train students in phonetic transcription.

CHAPTER

❸

The Teaching of Phonetic Transcription

A phonetic transcription is an impressionistic record of the phonetic properties of speech. In undertaking a phonetic transcription, one may wish to capture characteristics of individual speech segments (such as voice, place and manner of articulation for consonants) or aspects of longer stretches of speech (such as voice quality and intonation). This chapter looks at methods of training students to recognize and transcribe the phonetics of normal and disordered speech, with particular reference to segmental transcription. It also examines the relationship between transcription and other areas of phonetics and raises issues relevant to phonetics teaching and learning. These issues include accuracy and reliability in transcription and applicability of practice material that is presented to speech pathology students.

Transcription and General Phonetics

It needs to be recognized that students cannot become accomplished in phonetic transcription unless they are also proficient in other areas of phonetics. It is, therefore, naïve to assume that transcription can be taught or learned as an independent skill without reference to other areas. Some phonetics texts may, however, give the impression that transcription is a simple matter of matching a perceived sound with a written symbol. If this were the case, then transcription would amount to little more than a memory test. Listeners would merely need to remember that they need /θ/ to capture the first sound in *thin* and /tʃ/ to capture the first and last sounds in *church*, for example. The memory test approach may well be adequate for a broad transcription, but it is inadequate for a narrow one. For example, what happens if listeners perceive a sound that does not *quite* correspond to the written symbol stored in their mental dictionaries? The alveolar plosive in a standard American pronunciation of *computer*, for example may lack the completely voiceless feature associated with the target /t/ (hence [ˌkɒmˈpjuɾᵊr]), so that it may sound more like /d/. Cases such as this, in which the pronunciation of the sound varies somewhat from that of the general phoneme, may pose a problem for transcribers.

In normal and disordered speech, there are innumerable cases in which the characteristics of particular sounds differ substantially from those of their phonemic equivalents. In these cases, accurate phonetic transcription cannot be accomplished by simply matching sounds with symbols. A realistic transcription can be provided only when one can work out how the sound differs from its phonemic equivalent. This is done by detailed listening to ensure accurate perception of the sound, by reproducing it, and thereby establishing its articulatory composition.

To achieve competence in transcribing fine phonetic distinctions between sounds, as well as phonemic distinctions, listeners need skills in two other main areas, auditory phonetics and articulatory phonetics. In addition, speech pathologists are called to analyze aspects of connected speech and, for this purpose, an understanding of phonology is crucial (for a discussion of the range of skills needed for transcription see, for example, Bailey, 1985; Ladefoged, 1982, p. 32; Shriberg, Hincke, & Trost-Steffen, 1987).

Auditory phonetics has two clear applications to transcription. First, it trains learners in detailed listening and focuses their attention on individual speech sounds as part of the overall acoustic signal. This focus is important for speech pathologists, as they must have the ability to perceive abnormality in individual sounds; untrained listeners, on the other hand, may be unaccustomed to segmenting speech into its component sounds. Second, practice in auditory phonetics enables listeners to recognize and identify particular speech sounds and to perceive differences between one sound and another. This systematic attention to speech sounds and to variation among them is a necessary prerequisite to transcription.

Articulatory phonetics provides information on the articulatory makeup of speech sounds. As we have said above, this information is crucial for a detailed phonetic transcription. For example, if one wishes to capture an abnormal production of a given sound, one first needs to know how to analyze its articulatory characteristics (in terms of the position of the vocal organs and the nature of the airflow) before we can indicate the characteristics in transcription. One may wish to indicate, for example, that a given speaker produces the initial and final sound in *tight* with lip rounding (as in [tʷaɪtʷ]), which does not occur in normal speech, or that the medial sound in *cover* is produced with a wider stricture between the upper teeth and lower lip than is usual, resulting in a weaker than normal airflow (hence the approximant [ʋ] rather than the target fricative /v/). Without knowledge of articulatory features, the transcriber might not be able to work out these abnormalities, nor could they actually be indicated in transcription.

Finally, a comprehension of phonology makes an important contribution to transcription, particularly at the level of recording phonological processes in connected speech. For example, if listeners are aware that a phonological process such as insertion, for example, often operates in particular environments, then they are sensitized to such occurrences and will be able to transcribe them where necessary. In pronunciations of *dance* and *strength*, for example, speakers may optionally insert a sound between the nasal and the voiceless fricative, i.e. [dænts] and [stɹɛŋkθ]. Without an understanding of basic phonological processes, listeners may well fail to perceive and transcribe the inserted sound.

As well as optional phonological processes, there are of, course, several obligatory phonological processes in English, such as nasalization of a vowel preceding a nasal consonant (as in [bãnd]) and aspiration of a voiceless stop in word-initial stressed position (as in [tʰɒp]). It is arguable if information on obligatory phonological processes should be noted in transcription, on the grounds that it is predictable and, therefore, redundant. One should remember, however, that the predictability may not apply to disordered speech. Clinicians are, for instance, likely to encounter cases in which disordered speech does not follow the rules of typical English phonology. For example, we consider a patient who produces the final plosive in *asked* as a fully voiced sound, as in [askˀd]. This pronunciation would sound peculiar and the peculiarity can be accounted for by referring to the phonology of normal English. In normal speech, there is an assimilatory phonological process whereby a voiced obstruent following a voiceless obstruent becomes devoiced. The example above would therefore be realized as [askˀd̥], where the second stop assimilates to the voicelessness of the first. This process does not operate when *asked* is produced as [askˀd]. Our perception and explanation of phonological abnormality in disordered speech may, therefore, be aided by a detailed awareness of the phonology of normal speech. On these grounds, we suggest that familiarity with obligatory phonological processes should be encouraged, that they should be recorded in the transcription of both normal and disordered speech and their absence noted in disordered speech.

When speech pathology students possess well-developed skills in auditory and articulatory phonetics and phonology, they are in a position to produce a realistic transcription of the phonetic and phonological characteristics of disordered speech. At this point, we wish to comment briefly on the need for accurate transcription in assessing disordered speech. (This will be discussed in detail in Chapter 5.)

The Need for Accuracy in Transcription

To provide a valid assessment of disordered speech and to formulate a plan for therapy, then a reliable transcription is needed to begin with (the role of transcription in assessment is discussed by Bailey, 1985, for example). The central choice facing clinicians is whether to base the assessment on a phonemic or a phonetic transcription. A phonemic transcription can do no more than capture contrasts between major classes of sound and it is therefore successful in dealing with only a limited amount of data. It allows, for example, the capture of simple disorders such as errors in place of articulation (the substitution of a glottal plosive [ʔ] for the bilabial plosive /p/, see Howard, 1993), or errors in manner of articulation (the substitution of a plosive [p] for the target fricative /f/, see Grunwell & Russell, 1988). However, typically, errors are encountered that demand a narrower degree of analysis. For example, it may be needed to indicate that the target alveolar consonants /t/ and /d/ are produced with the tongue against the upper lip rather than against the alveolar ridge (hence the linguolabial [t̼] and [d̼]). In such cases, a narrow phonetic transcription is required to give a true picture of the disorder and we may need particular reference to the Extensions to the International Phonetic Alphabet known as "ExtIPA" (the resources of extIPA for transcribing disordered speech are explained in detail in later chapters). Only when transcription is accurate (by which we mean that it captures all possible phonetic and phonological details of the speech), is it reasonable to use it as a basis for assessment.

One should not be sidetracked by the views of investigators who suggest that neither phonemic nor phonetic analysis is important in the assessment process. Siren and Wilcox (1990), for example, in a discussion of the utility of phonetic versus orthographic transcription methods, argue that transcription of speech sounds is unnecessary for most clinical and research purposes. They say that, "the information available in the orthographic transcription is sufficient for most purposes of language analysis in a clinical setting" (p. 138). Clearly, an orthographic transcription is adequate for syntactic and semantic assessment and investigators may be able to indicate simple disorders in phonology by orthographic means. The substitution of [g] for /k/ in word initial position could, for example, be indicated orthographically, as in *gar* and *gat* for *car* and *cat*. Nevertheless, orthography simply has no role in detailed phonetic analysis. This point is made by Evershed-Martin (1989) in a discussion of the necessity of using phonetic transcription to assess speech production.

> In assessment investigators draw on their understanding of phonetics, without which they would be ill equipped to describe, identify and classify speech, or to judge anything but the most obvious errors. (p. 50)

So far in this chapter, we have established two main points important for transcribing the phonetics of disordered speech. These are that transcription skills require competence in various areas of phonetics and that transcription must be accurate if it is to be a worthwhile tool in speech pathology.

We now move on to look at some ways in which teachers may equip students with the skills necessary to produce an accurate transcription. First, we review a range of teaching and learning materials and assess the usefulness of practice transcription material that has traditionally been presented to speech pathology students. We then look briefly at some topics which may be of interest to those involved in screening potential students for phonetic ability and explore explanations for variation in ability. We do not intend this as a guide to identifying expert phonetics students, but merely as a presentation of some relevant issues. Finally, we highlight the need for reliability in transcription and suggest ways in which teachers can monitor reliability.

Materials for Teaching and Learning Phonetic Transcription

This section reviews a range of resources that can be used to teach and learn skills in phonetic transcription, from beginners' level through to more advanced stages. We look at books, audiotapes and videotapes, and computer software packages. Some of these materials are directly concerned with teaching transcription skills, but these are in the minority. Most resources target a range of phonetic abilities, in that they focus on auditory perception and articulatory description. By enhancing performance in auditory and articulatory phonetics, these materials have an important contribution to make to transcription. The majority of the resources reviewed here are designed for studying normal speech. Nevertheless, they could advantageously be adopted as elements of speech pathology courses, as they provide a solid grounding in the phonetics of normal speech which is vital for assessing disordered speech. Speech pathologists need to judge what is normal and what lies outside the bounds of normality and an informed understanding of normal speech will help them make the distinction.

Books

It is difficult to learn phonetics, whether auditory, articulatory, or transcriptional, from a book. However efficient the explanations, descriptions, and transcriptions of phonetic features contained therein, students need to hear speech sounds if they are to acquire competence in phonetics, and a book cannot reproduce the sounds of speech. When students are introduced to a sound, they should be able to hear it, should be able to reproduce it, and feel as well as understand its articulatory makeup. Phonetics teaching and learning should be in the context of constant aural stimulation; in summary, it should not be book-bound.

Nevertheless, a book is a useful component of a phonetics course. Its role is principally as a source of reference on the main areas of phonetic study, particularly articulatory descriptions of all sounds and explanations of the phonology of speech, with some reference to suprasegmentals and acoustic phonetics. This written information should be seen as complementary, rather than alternative, to information presented in the classroom and to aural training. We might, for example, envisage a situation in which a teacher introduces a concept such as vowel length and then directs students to the relevant portion of a book for detailed independent study of short and long vowels in English.

Most undergraduate textbooks in phonetics, whether American or British, cover similar core areas, in that they explain the production of speech sounds and their articulatory characteristics and provide examples of sound-letter correspondences as an introduction to transcription. Among those that have been favored in the past are K. L. Pike (1945), Smalley (1963), Abercrombie (1967), Malmberg (1968), O'Connor (1973), Wells and Colson (1973), Catford (1977), Ladefoged (1982), and Gimson (1989). Some of these also look at phonological processes of connected speech such as assimilation, insertion, deletion, and elision and explain suprasegmental aspects of connected speech such as rhythm, stress and intonation. In both of these respects, the texts by Wells and Colson and Gimson are particularly helpful. All of the texts aim to train students to a reasonable degree of phonemic transcription, so that they could transcribe broad differences between RP and General American pronunciation (such as ['lɑːgə] versus ['lɑːgər], for example, in which the presence or absence of postvocalic /r/ presents little problem for inexperienced transcribers) but not finer differences resulting from optional phonological voicing, (*mitreing* ['maɪtərɪŋ] in RP versus ['maɪ̮tərɪŋ] in General American is one instance of this). Most texts point out that there may be a wide variety of realizations of a single phoneme (O'Connor, 1973, for example, suggests an alternative [ɑ̈] realization for the usual [æ̈] in an RP pronunciation of *hat*), but none of the cited texts are concerned with training students to that degree of phonetic transcription. A minority of textbooks looks briefly at acoustic phonetics, but they are not intended as course books in acoustics.

With a small number of exceptions, the available books are intended for studying the phonetics of normal speech, although, as we have said above, these provide essential information for the speech pathology student. The teacher may, for example, choose to use these as preliminary texts and to provide additional information on abnormal speech from other sources, such as research papers. On the other hand, it may be more convenient to choose a text designed specifically for studying disordered speech. We now cover a selection of the most influential textbooks which are currently used in phonetics teaching in America and Britain.

In America, much introductory phonetics material occurs in general linguistics texts rather than in phonetic-specific form. To date, one of the most efficient presentations occurs in *Language Files*, edited by Jannedy, Poletto and Weldon, published by Ohio State University and now in a 1994 sixth edition. It begins with an introduction to English orthography and phonetic transcription, offering sound-letter correspondences for consonants and vowels. This initial focus on transcription is valuable; it immediately alerts learners that they can use phonetics as a tool to record their impressions of speech sounds. Most texts, on the other hand, introduce phonetics by explaining the physiological basis of speech production. Although information on the organs of speech is indispensable for speech pathologists, students may prefer the early concentration on transcription offered by *Language Files*, as it identifies one clear application of phonetics to their trade.

Language Files continues to sustain interest in transcription as a major pursuit in phonetics by providing inventive material for practice transcription (including passages from Woody Allen's book *Without Feathers*, for example). Much of the practice material provides the opportunity for two-way transcription, that is either from orthography into phonetics or vice versa. The ability to convert phonetic transcription into orthography is not one that is usually targeted by introductory textbooks. Nevertheless, it is a worthwhile skill. Most obviously, it increases familiarity with phonetic symbols and it likely has the added advantage of encouraging learners to convert their own phonetic transcriptions as a check on their accuracy. It is our impression that many student transcribers lack a critical awareness of their own transcriptions. They may feel that the task of finding symbols for sounds is taxing enough, without having to translate them back again. Nevertheless, training in translating from symbols to sounds should provide the opportunity for students to self-correct errors, thereby increasing accuracy in transcription.

The book provides an explanation of vowel theory that will appeal to instructors and learners in phonetics. As we have said above, an understanding of the articulatory characteristics of any speech sound is needed for accurate transcription. On the one hand, students usually manage to comprehend the articulatory makeup of consonants quickly. This may be because it is relatively easy to feel the points of contact or approximation of the articulators at fixed points along their own vocal tracts. During the production of vowels, however, it is more difficult to identify tongue activity in the oral cavity. Although Cardinal Vowel Theory offers the means of classifying articulatory characteristics, beginners in phonetics often have difficulty relating the theory to their own production of vowels in terms of frontness, backness, and vowel height. If this difficulty occurs, there is a danger that students will fall into the memory-test approach (see above), remembering that /ɔ/, for example, is a mid-open, back, rounded vowel, without being able to feel its location in their oral cavity. This will clearly pose difficulties when they need to transcribe a vowel that differs in some fine respects from Cardinal Vowel 6. Some southern American pronunciations of *boys*, for example, contain a diphthong whose starting point is lower than the position of Cardinal Vowel 6 ([bʔɪz]). The explanation of vowel theory in *Language Files* (Jannedy et al., 1994) offers a simple way of relating the theory to production, by presenting the usual vowel trapezium within a schematic mid-sagittal section of the oral cavity (see Figure 3–1).

It has been noted elsewhere (see Ball, 1993, p. 73) that vowel systems are largely ignored in studies of disordered speech. One simple explanation for this neglect might be that the theory of vowel production is often poorly understood. Teachers can address the situation by contextualizing vowel theory by relating the theory to tongue activity in a way that students can visualize and understand. The representation offered by *Language Files* (Jannedy et al., 1994) offers a systematic means of doing so. When students understand how the theoretical description relates to their own articulatory vowel space, they are in a position to record fine details in vowel differences in transcription.

An introductory phonetics text by Rogers (1991) is directed primarily at the Canadian market. As well as the basic material on classifying speech sounds, it contains a discussion of the vowel and consonant differences between Canadian English, American English, and RP plus a chapter on French, concentrating on Canadian French. Each chapter ends with exercises designed to test readers' understanding of the material presented. Two features of the book are unusual for introductory phonetics texts: its detailed introduction to acoustic phonetics (including detailed analyses of spectrograms) and its extensive treatment of phonological theory.

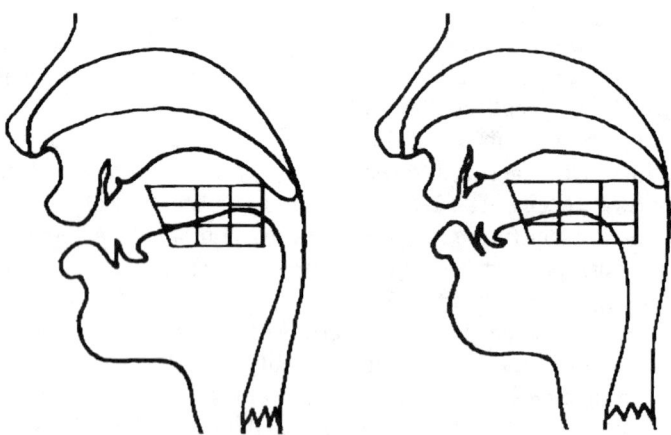

Figure 3–1. Mid-sagittal section of the oral cavity from *Language Files.*

In Britain, a range of texts on general elementary phonetics has been used at undergraduate level in the past (see those mentioned above). Although these contain much material of continuing value, they have three main drawbacks that may render them inappropriate as present-day course texts. First, they concentrate on describing the phonetics of rather formal varieties of speech; second, they contain rather little on the phonology of connected speech, and third, they offer little systematic advice for transcribing suprasegmental aspects of speech (although the material contained in Gimson, 1989, is helpful in the last respect). However, speech pathologists are increasingly called to transcribe informal speech, to capture the phonology of speech, and to comment in detail on its suprasegmental characteristics. It is likely, therefore, that they would wish for a text providing information on these topics.

Currently, the texts by Roach (1991) and Knowles (1987) are used in many British introductory courses, although neither claims to be a specialist book for producing phoneticians. Roach aims largely at "people learning English spoken in England" (p. 3) and Knowles at "students of linguistics or literature, teachers of English, and those involved with the study of literacy, or the analysis of discourse or conversation" (p. ix). Many British courses on phonetics also cover a considerable amount of phonology and the set texts are often weighted in favor of phonology such as Carr (1993) and Kriedler (1989). These assume some knowledge of phonetics or, at least, assume that such knowledge can be acquired quickly. They, therefore, begin with just a brief review of phonetic symbols and articulatory classifications of vowels and consonants. Clark and Yallop (1995), however, provide a text equally weighted in terms of introductory phonetics and phonology.

The most recent textbook on phonetics is Laver's (1994) *Principles of Phonetics*. This is the most comprehensive treatment of phonetics we have encountered and it will undoubtedly be chosen as the main text in phonetics courses in the future. All of the central issues in phonetics are covered and explained in a manner accessible to the beginner in phonetics and to the more advanced phonetician. One section of the book is entirely devoted to principles of transcription and the central discussion covers the distinction between phonemic and phonetic transcription. At a stage when most textbooks offer brief explanations of phonemic and phonetic transcription, equating them with "broad" and "narrow" analysis respectively,[1] Laver's focus represents a step forward in identifying the specific roles of particular transcription types.

With respect to phonetics texts intended directly for studying disordered speech, two texts are influential, Ball (1993) and M. L. Edwards (1986). These texts have two important advantages over the normal-based texts. First they pro-

---

[1]The relevance of the terms "broad" and "narrow" for transcription are detailed in Chapter 5.

vide a significant source of information on nonnormal sounds. Second, they pay specific attention to accuracy in transcription. Although normal-based texts tend to aim for a reasonable phonemic transcription to capture the major sound distinctions in speech, these texts encourage students to aim for accurate phonetic transcription. Ball, for example, offers a detailed list of symbols for capturing a wide range of abnormal sounds (extIPA), and Edwards highlights the need for students to attain particular standards of accuracy in transcription at each stage of training. Both texts, therefore, emphasize the importance of accurate transcription in assessing disordered speech. In addition, Ball's text provides a central source of information on some of the major features in a range of disordered speech types.

Edwards's text is based on General American and is designed as an introductory course on phonetics for students of communication disorders and linguistics. The author states that her aim is to help students learn transcription, although the text concentrates on providing learners with auditory training. It, therefore, implicitly acknowledges the important role that auditory training has in transcription. It is essentially a laboratory workbook with accompanying audiotapes covering seven laboratory sessions: oral and nasal stop consonants, fricatives and affricates, liquids and glides, front and back vowels, central vowels and diphthongs, commonly used diacritics and suprasegmentals. Each session consists of a brief description of the sound types and demonstrations of the sound in real words. This is followed by a series of self-test exercises, using both real and nonsense words with answers supplied at the back of the book. Each session concludes with a test to be marked by the teacher.

One of the most useful features of the book is that Edwards provides targets of accuracy to aim for in transcription. She suggests that a score of 95% success in transcribing real words and 90% for nonsense words should be achieved in each exercise before students proceed to the next one. These targets are effective means of monitoring progress in transcription, both for teachers and for the students, themselves. The targets are also effective in impressing on students the need for accuracy in transcription.

In Britain, Ball's (1993) text is intended for students following courses in speech pathology and therapy. It consists of sections on articulatory, acoustic, and auditory phonetics, with each chapter linking theoretical aspects to speech problems of various types. For example, the chapter on vowels highlights a disruption to the vowel system (such as loss of vowel units or changes in the phonetic quality of vowels) that may well occur in disordered speech, but which is often ignored in studies of phonological disorders. The chapter on plosive theory discusses difficulties with the fine control needed to produce basic stop types (the example given illustrates difficulties with lateral and nasal release of stops, where epenthetic vowels are inserted between stops and nasals and stops and laterals, as in ['bʌtən] and ['mɪdəl] for ['bʌtn] and ['mɪdl]). Each chapter provides suggestions for further reading, which helps provide comprehensive coverage of the issues in question.

We do not wish to suggest that American and British texts are necessarily in opposition to one another. The division into British and American textbooks in this chapter is largely a convenient means of presenting texts favored on either side of the Atlantic and of highlighting texts that may be more readily available to students in either country. Of course, there may be problems with some phonetic symbols, insofar as American texts often use a distinct system of symbolization, and some keywords might be sources of difficulty. In *Language Files*, for example, the phonetic alphabet used varies in some respects from the IPA and the keywords given for the symbols may be confusing ([a] is given as the realization of the underlined vowel in p<u>o</u>t, h<u>o</u>nor, h<u>o</u>spital and mel<u>o</u>dic, for example). For these reasons, we imagine that American and British students may prefer American and British texts, respectively.

In short, there is a rather narrow range of textbooks in phonetics to choose from. One major decision facing the phonetics teacher is whether to adopt a book dealing with normal speech and to provide additional material on disordered speech from other sources or to adopt a text covering normal as well as disordered speech. For a dedicated speech pathology course, it would seem wise to choose the second alternative.

Audio Recordings

Audio recordings are a central component of phonetics learning. They offer intensive training in auditory perception, which, in turn, acts as important preparation for transcription. In the early stages of phonetics learning, students should be introduced to a system of aural training in the classroom. They should, for example, be guided to listen carefully to speech sounds, reproduce, label, and finally transcribe them. Having practiced these skills, students should then be able to apply them in their own independent listening and transcription practice, using recorded audiotape material as exercises.

Audiotapes for training auditory phonetics come from various sources. They may, for example, be prepared by the phonetics teacher, to give practice transcription at each stage of the course. For instance, a class on diacritics might be supplemented by a tape containing a reading passage produced with a range of accents. The students would then be directed to capture the differences among the accents by using diacritics as well as other appropriate means. They might have to indicate, for example, differences in the Australian versus the GenAm pronunciation of *fly*, in which case they would need diacritics to capture the raised and advanced opening element of the diphthong in the Australian pronunciation compared to the American one. If such tapes are used in conjunction with the language laboratory facilities, students would have the option of recording their own speech alongside the original version. They could compare their own production with the one on tape, thereby sharpening their perception and production skills even further. Student performance in such exercises should be monitored by the teacher to keep a check on progress and accuracy in transcription.

Other tapes are available commercially and fall into two main categories. Some are merely illustrative (such as "The Sounds of the International Phonetic Alphabet," produced by University College, London), although others both exemplify and provide practical test examples. Most of the tapes accompanying textbooks on phonetics fall into the second category (in the case of Edwards, 1986 and Roach 1991). When these tapes are used in combination with the textbooks, the authors aim at a self-contained course in phonetics. However, although the provision of some kind of auditory material to accompany a written text is to be recommended, such tapes do have drawbacks. In particular, they present rather formal varieties of speech and the examples tend to be somewhat short.

For audiotapes containing examples of disordered speech, in particular, individual colleges of speech therapy may be the best source (see, for example, those produced by Queen Margaret College, Edinburgh, UK). Although these tend not to offer formal test exercises in transcription, such tapes provide an invaluable opportunity for students to familiarize themselves with a range of disordered speech types. Teachers may, of course, wish to adapt taped material to test situations by directing students to prepare transcriptions of the audio material.

The most beneficial tapes for the speech and language pathology student are likely to be those devised by individual teachers and those produced by speech therapy colleges. Teacher-produced tapes are immediately relevant to students, as they reinforce issues as they are introduced in the classroom. Those prepared by speech therapy colleges offer possibilities for intensive exposure to and practice transcription of disordered speech. Although tapes that accompany textbooks may be helpful at a preliminary stage in phonetics for practice in broad transcription, they have a limited application for the speech pathology student.

Video Recordings

The video recordings that are of value in phonetics teaching and learning are of three kinds. First, there are those that provide x-ray photography of the vocal tract, showing glottal activity and the movement of the articulators during the production of oral and nasal sounds. An x-ray presentation of the tongue in the oral cavity provides an opportunity for students to relate tongue movement to vowel theory, so that they can see which part of the tongue forms the obstruction in any vowel and are then able to describe the articulatory characteristics of the vowel. These videos therefore aid students' understanding of the physiological processes underlying speech production and help them visualize the activity of the articulators.

Second, there are videos that help enhance perceptual phonetic skills by showing speakers producing a range of speech sounds. Those produced by the University of Edinburgh, U.K., for example, consist of units on phonation, consonants, palatals and palato-alveolars, central and lateral sounds, retroflex sounds, oral and nasal stops, double and secondary articulations and, finally, ejectives and implosives. One of the units specifically covers the visual clues to help auditory perception, for example in the case of bilabial and labiodental consonants /m/ and /ɱ/ respectively. As well as training in auditory perception, these videos, therefore, offer additional help in sound differentiation for sounds that differ little in their acoustic makeup.

The third type may be of less obvious use to phonetics learning. These are the videos that demonstrate instrumental techniques for phonetic study, and we wish to concentrate here on one videotape illustrating the technique of electropalatography (prepared by the Department of Linguistic Science at the University of Reading, U.K.). Electropalatography (EPG) is the method that records details of tongue contact with the palate during continuous speech (see Hardcastle, Jones, Knight, Trudgeon, & Calder, 1989, for a discussion of the technique). Figure 3–2 shows a sample video screen of normal and abnormal productions of the target /s/.

This kind of representation encourages learners to relate abnormal sounds to articulatory patterns and, as we have previously stated, this is likely to inform the transcription process. Although beginning phonetics students are clearly not expected to cover courses in EPG, a basic familiarity with the method and aims of EPG, such as provided by the Reading video, should help students become accustomed to recognizing fine differences among speech sounds.

These three types of video have an important role in phonetics training. They offer the chance for students to familiarize themselves in detail with the location and movement of the articulators, not merely from abstract charts and diagrams,

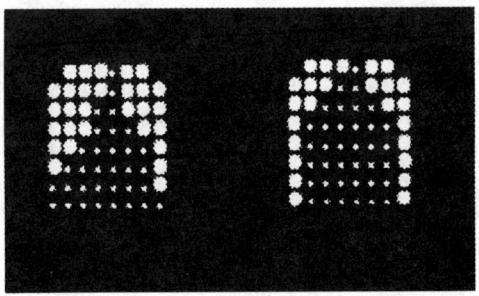

Figure 3–2. An electropalatographic trace.

but by means of visualization of the human vocal tract. This familiarity, along with training in auditory and visual perception allows listeners to learn to identify and describe phonetic contrasts.

Computer Software

Computer-based methods for teaching and learning phonetics constitute a major growth area in the subject. Although the listed books and tapes are essentially directed at students in individual and isolated study, computer programs in phonetics allow students to learn in an interactive environment, with the software package posing questions that the student answers and the software providing feedback by confirming or providing the answer if the student requires it. Software for phonetics training falls into two main categories. The first is general software, which trains in a range of phonetic skills, auditory perception and articulatory description as a prerequisite to transcription. The second category targets transcription skill directly. By far the majority of these packages deal with phonemic rather than phonetic transcription and with the transcription of normal speech.

General Phonetics Software Packages

These packages use similar methods to train students in auditory perception, transcription and articulatory description. Users are presented with digitized test sounds that they must first identify auditorily and then match with the appropriate IPA symbol. They then have the option of repeating the test sound several times and if they are still unable to identify it, the program will provide the answer.

The 1986 Phonetic Symbol Guide—Electronic Edition (PSG) is a Hyper-Card-based version of Pullum and Ladusaw's (1986) book *Phonetic Symbol Guide*. Neither the book nor the program is intended as an introduction to phonetics and each presupposes a grounding in phonetic theory. However, either could reasonably be incorporated early on in any phonetics course.

Although the book and the program contain the same information, the program has a number of clear advantages. First, it it allows users to *listen* to the sounds. Secondly, the program allows users more choice in how they approach particular topics. For example, the book is arranged by symbol, in that a user looks up unfamiliar symbols and then finds comprehensive guidance about their meaning. With the program, users may, on the one hand, choose to navigate the program in a similar symbol-based way. This symbol-based system, however, is a somewhat limited way of approaching the information contained in PSG. Users may, however, prefer to work systematically on general classes of sounds (consonants with the same place of articulation, or unrounded vowels, for example). The program therefore offers more flexibility in learning methods than the text. We should note, however, that as the program was prepared in 1986, it does not incorporate the 1989 revisions to particular IPA symbols.

A central feature of the program is that it provides exercises for users to discriminate sounds. Two exercises are provided, one for consonants and one for vowels (the screen for vowels is shown in Figure 3–3). In each case, users are presented with a test vowel that they can choose to hear again and again. Perception of the sound can be checked by clicking on any of the symbols on the screen and matching the test sound with one of them. Users can then confirm their identification by prompting the program to reveal the test symbol. At any stage, users can discover information about a symbol by clicking on a number of categories: "IPA usage," "American usage," "Other Uses," and "Comments and Sources."

PSG presents a variety of classificational systems for vowels and consonants. Vowels, for example, are divided into the IPA categories of primary and secondary cardinals and unrounded and rounded vowels. Bloch and Trager's (1942) vowel system is also represented, as is the Chomsky-Halle (1968) classification, along with standard American usage. Consonant charts are divided between obstruent, resonant and non-pulmonic sounds for both IPA and American usages and users can click any of the symbols on the charts to hear the symbol produced.

A second HyperCard-based program for learning phonetics, *The Sounds of the International Phonetic Alphabet* (no date given on the software) is rather less

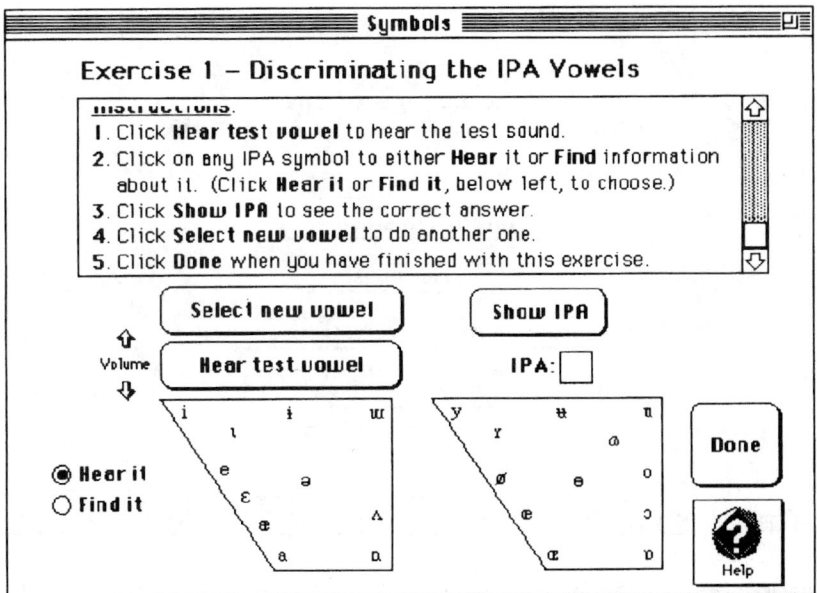

Figure 3–3. Vowel screen from "Phonetic Symbol Guide—Electronic Edition."

ambitious than PSG. It simply provides sounds for users to listen to and identify and does not attempt to provide detailed information on the theoretical side of phonetics. The program consists of four main sections: nasals and plosives; fricatives; approximants, laterals, trills and taps; non-pulmonic sounds, and vowels. Figure 3–4 shows the opening menu in the program, divided into these sections.

Furthermore, the sounds are not presented in charts as in PSG, but according to place of articulation, with left to right corresponding to the progression from bilabial to glottal places (where possible). Figure 3–5 shows the presentation for nasals and plosives. Clicking on any symbol will play a recording of that sound and clicking on "Quiz" will select a random sound that is then played. As was the case with PSG, users can check their impressions by comparing the test sound with any of those displayed on the screen. They can then prompt the software to display the correct symbol, along with its accompanying articulatory description, by clicking on the "Answer" box.

In addition, two non HyperCard-based programs are in preparation that have potentially valuable applications to phonetics teaching. Nicholas Reid from the University of New England, Australia, is currently developing an interactive phonetics package using Photoshop and Authorware software. The package includes IPA symbols for all Australian English consonants, for cardinal vowels (all primary and some secondary), and Australian English vowels. Students will have the opportunity for self-testing exercises in all of these categories. The package includes a vocal tract diagram, which will allow users to click on labeled

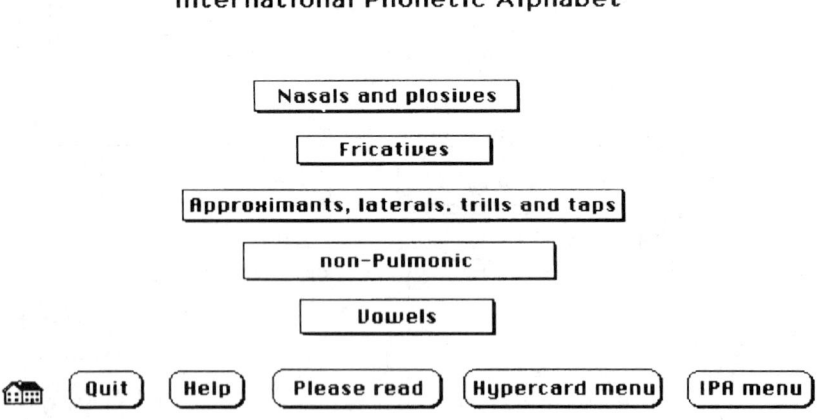

Figure 3–4. Opening menu from "The Sounds of the International Phonetic Alphabet."

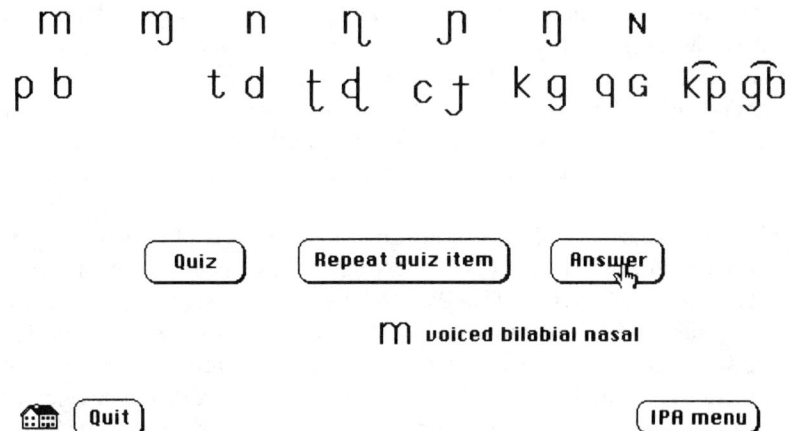

Figure 3-5. Nasals and plosives section from "The Sounds of the International Phonetic Alphabet."

organs and find out some information about them. A further package is being prepared by Ian Smith from York University, U.K. He intends to produce a multimedia phonetics resource running under Windows; it will consist of digitized video clips of a speaker demonstrating individual sounds, together with software to access these clips in a variety of ways by means of, for one example, tutorials on particular sound classes.

As we have noted, the general software packages offer an important input to phonetic transcription. By training students in auditory and articulatory phonetics, their perception is enhanced, and it therefore acts as an aid to transcription. We now look at the packages specifically designed for training in transcription.

Transcription Oriented Packages

The transcription oriented packages that are available vary enormously in sophistication. Even the least ambitious packages, however, offer useful exercises in transcription. One of these is called *PHONETICS* (devised in 1991) and it provides simple exercises for transcribing RP phonetics in particular. It runs on any machine with MS DOS 3.3 or later equipped with EGA video or better and there is also a version for the Amstrad PCW. The software reads in a file of word and transcription pairs, and presents them in either direction: it can present an orthographic word to be transcribed into phonetics or a phonetically transcribed word to be identified. When the exercise is transcription into phonetics, the screen displays a plan of all the possible characters and their location on the keyboard. If a user enters an illegal character (such as a capital letter) the machine beeps. Feedback when the exercise is finished is rather crude: performance is assessed as right, not quite right and not right. A new version, however, is expected to pinpoint errors within the word. Users are permitted three chances before the software provides the right answer. The software also offers a simple editor for creating new exercises, which may be of interest to teachers wishing to design their own tests.

A more advanced facility for transcription learning is provided by the phonetics component of the HyperText collection. It presents users with a transcription of Edward Lear's poem "The Owl and the Pussy Cat," with each line containing a clear mistake in transcription. Users can check their recognition of phonetic symbols by clicking on what they think are the mistakes. The computer will respond by telling them whether their selection is correct or not. One particularly useful feature is that the package also shows transcriptions of different accents of the poem. This last feature sensitizes students from an early stage that differences in pronunciation should be reflected in transcription.

By far the most impressive computerized aid to transcription is the IPA Transcription Tutorial (discussed in detail in Chapter 9), Model 4335 program running on the Kay Computerized Speech Lab™ (CSL). The program is designed to help students of phonetics, linguistics and speech science to learn and use the IPA. Although it contains the capabilities of the more basic programs mentioned above (students can click on symbols and hear them produced), it also offers more exciting possibilities. For example, it aids transcribers in assigning IPA symbols to their own data. If transcribers are in doubt as to which sound is being used in a given stretch of speech, they can call up stored sampled sounds along with their spectrographic and palatographic displays and compare them with the sound in question. At present, the CSL Tutorial Program only covers normal speech, but the program is currently being extended to include symbols for the transcription of disordered speech. (This is discussed in detail in Chapter 9.)

In summary, a wide range of materials is available to supplement classroom activity. Textbooks provide a source of reference, audio and video material enhances perceptual skills, and computer packages provide an interactive learning environment. Computer software has an important role to play, because it allows students to progress largely at their own rate, they receive immediate feedback on their progress, and the interactive learning possibilities provide them with stimulus for independent study when they are not in the classroom. In one sense, the software packages combine the best of books and audio materials by offering information and sound in one location. Although not all of these materials target transcriptional skills directly, it is suggested here that the skills they do encourage are vital to accurate transcription.

Relevance of Practice Transcription Material

Speech pathologists in clinics are likely to encounter a range of speech types that they must transcribe. Consider, for example, a patient presenting with a particular speech disorder unfamiliar to the pathologist, combined with an unfamiliar accent or even language background. As far as possible, student pathologists should be prepared for such eventualities by training in relevant material. By "relevant," we mean speech from a range of accent backgrounds, both normal and disordered, and from a variety of speech styles, formal and informal. Of course, it is impossible to prepare students for all clinical eventualities, but they should at least have some experience of transcribing nonfamiliar speech sounds, for example in nonsense words and foreign languages.

Much material giving guidance on transcription leaves the impression that speakers usually use relatively formal RP or GenAm and that they produce cardinal vowels most of the time. Although sociolinguistics has long recognized that speech varies according to a wide range of factors, such as formality and social class background, this information has largely failed to influence guides to phonetics learning. The result is that students are often expert phonemic listeners (see Ball, 1993, p. 209), but they may be at a loss when it comes to transcribing anything other than the broad phonemes of the speech in question. One consequence of phonemic listening is that listeners may transcribe what they expect to hear, rather than the sound that is, in fact, uttered. In the clinical context, such a possibility is dangerous, as clinicians may identify as abnormal a usage that simply reflects community norms. In some varieties of Irish English, for example, *sixth* is acceptably realized as [sɪkst], but lack of familiarity with this pronunciation may lead a listener to classify it as abnormal. To attempt to overcome such eventualities, speech pathology students should be presented with data that reflects language variation in unfamiliar backgrounds, as well as data covering a range of phonological variation in their native communities.

In clinical assessment of speech, the role of language variation in relation to communicative context is particularly important (see W. Wells, 1994). There are, for example, reports of intonation in the speech of patients who are postlingually deafened sounding hyperformal in informal contexts and vice versa (Rahilly, 1991). This stylistic inappropriateness may extend to the realization of individual segments and lead to the speakers being misunderstood or perceived as difficult in particular circumstances. If therapists wish to provide training for patients that will enhance their communication skills (Samar & Metz, 1991, and Smith 1975, for example, state that this is a major goal of therapy), then they need to assess speech in relation to a range of communicative situations, to target all possible contexts in which speech is likely to be disordered. This focus on the communicative and interactive aspects of clinical activity has been shown to be important (see Crystal, 1984) and we are now familiar with terms such as "clinical pragmatics," "clinical discourse analysis" (Crystal, 1984) and "clinical sociolinguistics" (Ball, 1992). All assessment situations therefore, need to take account of phonetic variation in relation to a range of communicative contexts.

Although it is clearly desirable that all transcribers should be exposed to speech from a range of accent and language and stylistic backgrounds, it is a fundamental requirement for those involved in assessing disordered speech.

Variety in Phonetic Ability Among Students

Given the large numbers of applicants for places in speech pathology courses and the small number of places available, institutions may need to be highly selective in choosing students. The selection process may involve some screening for potential phonetic ability. In the screening situation, it will come as no surprize that there is enormous variation in ability. Shriberg et al. (1987) for example, made the point neatly:

> Every phonetician must have had the experience, at some time or other of meeting a person to whom the imitation of the most exotic sounds at first hearing presented no difficulty at all. At the other extreme are a more numerous minority who are hopelessly recalcitrant, and for whom any deviation from the native sound system is apparently impossible. (p. 91)

Similarly, Rosenthal (1989) states that many students need considerable amounts of practice, drill, and feedback with multiple examples before they reach an acceptable standard. Ladefoged (1982), with particular reference to the teaching of implosives, says that, "some people can learn to make them by just imitating their instructor; others can't" (p. 123).

It can be helpful for instructors to pinpoint some variables that are known to contribute to phonetic ability. The literature makes some general suggestions about the relationship between phonetic ability and external variables and although the relationships make intuitive sense, they are far from systematically proven. Nevertheless, we will briefly outline them here. Shriberg et al. (1987), for example, speculate about the role that a musical background has to play as a predictor of phonetic competence. They say:

> Although we suspect it is neither a necessary nor a sufficient predictor variable. . . , most of our transcribers with really good ears have had a substantial background as instrumentalists. (p. 182)

Strevens (1978) also highlights a range of factors that may affect phonetics learning, such as variation in willingness to learn, variations in greater or less possession of a "good ear," normally taken to mean good auditory discrimination together with greater alertness of hearing.

Not surprisingly, phonetics is comparable to any other discipline, insofar as there are both relatively fast and slow learners. Some appreciation of the factors that may be likely to play a role in phonetic ability, however, may be helpful in selecting students when places are at a premium.

Reliability in Transcription

Teachers need to ensure that there is a high degree of reliability among student transcriptions. It is important that reliability is monitored continually, from the earliest stages in phonetics learning, so that students do not fall into the habit of producing mediocre transcriptions. Reliable transcriptions are clearly of central importance in clinical assessment. Kearns and Simmons (1988) for instance, call for specialized training in this area and point out that little systematic attention has been paid to the issue of reliability in transcription. Even among trained transcribers, however, agreement in transcription may not be high. Shriberg and Lof (1991), for example, reported agreements ranging from 28% to 58% in transcriptions of a series of continuous speech utterances from young children with moderately to severely delayed speech development. When agreements between transcribers are particularly low, transcribers attempt to solve the problem by choosing the most objectively acceptable transcription (this is known as the consensus procedure). It is unlikely that teachers will have the available time to monitor reliability between transcribers in a systematic and detailed manner. Nevertheless, it should be possible to select small pieces of data, prepared by different transcribers, for comparison. The teacher can, for example, point out errors in transcription and suggest the correct version or compare alternative transcriptions and attempt to arrive at objectively acceptable transcriptions by consensus.

In this chapter, we have discussed a range of material and methods of value for teaching and learning phonetic transcription, from introductory through to more advanced stages. Chapter 4 looks in detail at the phonetic characteristics of disordered speech that have to be recorded in transcription.

CHAPTER

4

Transcription and Disordered Speech

There is a wide range of disordered speech, resulting in a great variety of atypical and nonnormal phonetic characteristics that may need to be described. This description has, of course, been mainly in the form of impressionistic transcription, although in recent times instrumental analyses have become more common. Even here, these accounts generally associate instrumental findings with a phonetic transcription.

Traditionally, the IPA has been the transcription system favored by speech pathologists and clinical phoneticians on both sides of the Atlantic, even considering the practice within American linguistics of using the U.S. transcription system discussed in Chapter 1. This means that speech pathology in the U.S. is firmly within the international community for phonetic description.

Serious examination of the phonetics of speech disorders dates from around the time that phoneticians began to codify a symbol system for phonetic description—the last quarter of the nineteenth century (see Chapter 1). It is not surprising, therefore, that the IPA has been an essential part of speech pathology courses in most centers for many years. However, there are areas in which the use of the IPA needs clarification and there are others in which the IPA may not be sufficient for the task of describing disordered speech. We address these points in this chapter.

Phonetic Versus Phonological Transcription

As noted in Chapter 2, it is perfectly feasible to use either a phonetic or phonological (i.e., phonemic) transcription system. The two procedures have different goals: a detailed description of all the sounds used or an analysis of the use of the contrastive sound units of the particular language. The question that arises with disordered speech is which of these two approaches should be used in transcription.

Quite clearly, one of the main reasons why certain speech is labeled disordered is because the normal organization into contrastive sound units has broken down and so the speaker cannot be said to be using the expected phonological system. This is true whether the disorder has resulted in a disruption to the phonemic or to the allophonic level of description. In such an event, then, it would not seem very sensible to attempt a transcription based on the phonological/phonemic level. One surely needs as much phonetic information as possible (from which, if desired, one can build up a picture of the patient's own phonological system), and this means that only a detailed phonetic transcription has any validity with disordered speech.

This particular point will be returned to in more detail in the next chapter, where we will attempt to illustrate some of the pitfalls that can result from relying on a "broad" phonemic transcription, instead of a "narrow" phonetic one.

Aspects of Disordered Speech

When considering the phonetics of disordered speech, we can either examine in turn a variety of speech disorders and their phonetic manifestations, or examine a variety of phonetic features and see in what ways they may be manifested in disordered speech that are different from normal speech. As certain phonetic characteristics are found in a variety of speech disorders, we would be at-risk of continuous repetition if we took the first option. Therefore, in this chapter we examine disordered speech from the phonetic end rather than in terms of the specific disorder.

We will divide our description into three main categories: consonants, vowels, and prosodic features (also termed suprasegmentals). We are not interested here in phonological aspects such as disruptions to phonemes or to the phonotactics of a language, as such matters are beyond the scope of this book.

We must also bear in mind that what may seem a disordered pronunciation for the speaker of English, may be a quite ordinary consonant or vowel in another language. In most of these instances, we have perfectly satisfactory symbolization available in the IPA, and such sounds should cause no difficulty to the well-trained transcriber. What we are interested in mainly in this chapter are the sounds that are only very rarely encountered in natural language, or sounds that are never so encountered and are restricted to particular speech disorders and for which the IPA has no symbols. The IPA chart revised in 1993 is reproduced in Appendix 1 (IPA, 1989, 1993).

Consonants

If we consider the full list of descriptive parameters we can use in describing consonants (as in Ball, 1993, p. 82, for example, although we do not follow the same order of features here), we can approach possible atypical consonant productions from those categories.

Airstream Mechanism and Direction

Although speech is usually expected to be produced on a pulmonic egressive airstream, we know that it is possible to use other airstreams. Some of these are found in natural language (velaric ingressive and glottalic egressive and ingressive) and there are IPA symbols for these. Some, however, are not so found, and particularly one might think of pulmonic ingressive speech (found, for example, in the speech of some disfluent patients) and speech using air belched from the stomach through the esophagus. This latter, often termed esophageal speech, is commonly found in patients who have undergone laryngectomy. Neither pulmonic ingressive speech nor esophageal speech can be denoted in the IPA.

Phonation

The two phonation types used linguistically in English are the voiced and voiceless types. (Other phonation types can be found, generally over longer stretches of speech than a single segment and so these are covered under prosodic features below.) It is, of course, quite easy to mark which consonants are voiced and which voiceless through the use of the relevant symbols; but there are some instances where this may not be sufficient. We may wish to transcribe a voiceless consonant where the IPA only provides a symbol for the voiced equivalent (e.g. with nasals and liquids). In this case one can employ the under-ring diacritic as in [n̥], [l̥]. We may also wish to illustrate in our transcription finer degrees of voicing information, such as devoicing at the beginning or end of an otherwise voiced segment or, conversely, partial voicing during some part of an otherwise voiceless segment. Inability to manipulate the voicing contrast of the target language may occur in a variety of speech disorders, ranging from developmental disorders through to acquired neurological disorders.

Connected with phonation is aspiration. Although the IPA clearly marks the presence of aspiration through the superscript-h (e.g. [pʰ]), it does not have an overt marking for absence of aspiration. Although it might be argued that the absence of something need not be marked, it is clear the plain voiceless plosive symbols are so often used (phonemically, for example) in an "aspiration-neutral" manner, that such an extra diacritic might well be most useful to transcribe disordered speech and to mark that an expected aspirated segment was, in fact, unaspirated. We might also wish to have a means of marking pre-aspiration: that is to say, a period of voicelessness preceding the stop closure.

Strength of Articulation

The terms "fortis" and "lenis" (or "strong" and "weak") have long been used in the phonetic literature, although there has not always been agreement as to precisely what they mean. From a phonetic viewpoint, one normally considers strong sounds to be those that have used a greater degree of muscular effort (both in initiation and articulation) and normally a greater amount of airflow (and so will be perceived as louder). There have never been any diacritics in the IPA to mark this distinction as, by and large, voiceless sounds are considered fortis and voiced ones lenis. Even in the absence of full voicing or complete voicelessness, the choice by the transcriber of a "voiced" or a "voiceless" symbol was considered sufficient to mark whether the sound was to be understood as fortis or lenis.

However, in various types of speech disorder (e.g., disfluent speech, apraxic speech) we quite often encounter consonant productions that are stronger than would ever be found in normal speech (e.g. after a block in disfluent speech) or weaker than would normally be found in normal speech. We should be looking, therefore, for a means of marking such extra-fortis or extra-lenis articulations.

Place of Articulation

Clearly, if a patient uses a place of articulation different from the one expected for a specific consonant, it may well be a place for which the IPA provides symbols or diacritics. For example, if one finds the use of alveolar sounds instead of velar ones, there will be no difficulty in transcribing them. However, there is a range of places of articulation for consonants that are not found in natural language (or are extremely rare), but which are reported sufficiently often in clinics. For these, therefore, some means of transcription is clearly needed.

Included in this latter range would be articulations in the labial area: linguolabials (tongue tip to upper lip), labio-dental plosives (for which the IPA lacks symbols), dento-labials (i.e., reverse labio-dentals: upper lip and lower teeth), labio-alveolars (lower lip articulating with the alveolar lip, restricted probably to speakers with marked overbites). Clinical phoneticians also need to transcribe interdental articulations: that is, articulations that are not simply dental (with the tongue tip behind the upper front teeth), but actually have tongue tip protrusion between the upper and lower front teeth to a greater or lesser extent. Sounds of many manners of articulation can be made in this fashion; and indeed, the upper and lower teeth can be approximated even when non-tongue-tip sounds are involved, and can themselves be brought sharply together in a "percussive" manner to produce a consonant-like sound (percussives can also be produced by bringing the upper and lower lips together sharply). All of these dental features should be able to be transcribed. Places of articulation at the pharyngeal end of the vocal tract have also been described as occurring in disordered speech. We will return shortly to the so-called "velopharyngeal snort," but can note that both voiced and voiceless pharyngeal plosives were reported in PRDS (1983), although Laufer (1991) claims a voiced pharyngeal plosive is impossible to produce. It is quite possible that these were, in fact, epiglottal stops, and the current IPA has a symbol for an epiglottal stop. Nevertheless, we will list the PRDS suggestions for these stops later.

There is also the possibility that the place of articulation for a single segment in disordered speech will not be stable. As reported, for example, in Bernhardt and Ball (1993), some patients seem to utilize a "sliding" place of articulation, in that the articulator moves from one place to a neighboring one within the confines of a single segment. Clearly such behavior might well be of interest as a sign of possible system change and, again, one should be able to note this. This feature is not the same as double articulation: where two independent strictures are held in place at separate locations for the duration of the segment. These types are, of course, well known in natural language, and indeed [w] is usually defined as a labio-velar double articulation. However, one needs to be aware that less usual double articulation types (such as labio-alveolar or alveolo-velar stops) may well occur in clinical data. This point is returned to later.

Finally, we can consider the case of alveolar place of articulation. The IPA (1989, 1993) charts provide common symbols for most manners of articulation for dental, alveolar, and post-alveolar, with the general idea that if one wishes to specify dental place, one uses the dental diacritic and if one wishes to specify post-alveolar place, one uses the retraction diacritic. There is, however, no alveolar diacritic. This means that a plain symbol either stands for alveolar or for "unspecified: any of the three," depending, we are to suppose, on how detailed a transcription one is reading. This is clearly not satisfactory, and an unambiguous alveolar diacritic is clearly a desideratum. Further, as has been shown above, one may wish to specify articulations such as labio-alveolar, where the use of an alveolar diacritic could simplify the choice of transcription. Also, as will be shown in the upcoming section on prosodic features, a voice quality type such as "alveolarized voice" will require a specific diacritic to distinguish it from other voice qualities. We will look at the current proposal for such an alveolar diacritic and how it can be used.

Manner of Articulation

As one might expect, unlike place, there are not many novel, atypical manners of consonant articulation. An important feature that does seem to fit into this category is reiteration. The rapid repetition of segments or of syllables with no noticeable pausing is commonly encountered in disordered speech of various types (e.g., stuttering, but also various types of acquired neurogenic disorders) and is, indeed, found in the speech of nondisordered speakers to a greater or lesser extent. There has not been, however, any consistent method of marking such repetitions, and to distinguish between reiteration and other forms of repetition in which there are measurable (albeit very short) pauses between the repeated items. Clearly, an adequate transcription of a speaker with this kind of reiterative behavior requires an agreed symbolization.

A less important manner type that might require a notation is whistled fricative articulation. Typically occurring with apical fricatives, some speakers may produce such a narrowed fricative groove that the resulting air flow produces a whistle rather than a normal fricative. This type of sound is generally thought of as atypical, although it can occur in the speech of those otherwise characterized as normal speakers. Nevertheless, a symbol is needed to denote this articulation type.

Central Versus Lateral Articulation

In normal speech phoneticians are used to describing consonants in terms of whether the release of the air flow is central over the tongue or lateral over the side rims of the tongue. Indeed, one can specify in the latter case whether the lateral release was unilateral (over one side of the tongue: "dexter" [right] or "sinister" [left]), or bilateral (over both sides), although this rarely presents as a perceptible difference. Certain types of lisp in child speech disorders involve the transfer of target central fricatives (such as [s, z] or [ʃ, ʒ]) to lateral fricatives ([ɬ, ɮ]).

However, this is not the whole story. There are also instances of lisps where the resultant fricative has both central and lateral release. By this we mean that there is a channel made centrally allowing some air to be released along the middle of the tongue, but there is also (usually a unilateral) channel at the side of the tongue, allowing some lateral release of air. Such articulations are shown well on electropalatographic equipment (see Hardcastle & Gibbon, in press). Clearly, terms such as "lateral lisp" or "lateralization" (frequently encountered in the speech pathology literature) are unclear and misleading here, as they do not distinguish between these two types of articulation. "Lateralization" is particularly unfortunate because, if we look at the similar sounding terms, "palatalization," "velarization," and so on, it would suggest a secondary lateral aspect, when it is clear that it is normally employed to denote the change from central target fricative to lateral realization. It would be much better to use terms such as "lateral fricative" and "central-lateral fricative" in such cases. At any rate, it is clear a set of symbols to denote both voiced and voiceless central-lateral fricatives is needed.

Nasality/Orality

Symbols for normal speech can help distinguish among three degrees of nasality/orality: nasal—with air flow solely out of the nasal cavity; oral—in which air flows solely out of the oral cavity; and nasalized—with air flow out of the nasal cavity and oral cavity simultaneously. For nasal the relevant nasal consonant symbol (e.g., [m, n, ŋ, ɲ, ɴ]) is employed; for oral the relevant oral consonant symbol is employed; and for nasalized we add the nasalization diacritic (or tilde) to an oral symbol (e.g., [ṽ, r̃)]).

However, in disordered speech—particularly when velo-pharyngeal inadequacy is involved—other types and degrees of nasality (or indeed loss of nasality) may be found that need to be transcribed. For example, the current IPA provides no way of marking denasalized sounds. Although one might imagine that denasalized simply requires the use of the non-nasal (i.e., oral symbol), one may well wish to recognize that a particular nasal target is pronounced with a degree of nasality noticeably less than normal (i.e., not totally oral) and for such purposes the use of an oral symbol is not well motivated.

Another category phoneticians might well wish to mark in a transcription is that of audible nasal airflow, or nasal friction. Whereas a nasal stop such as [m] or [n], or a nasalized vowel such as [ã] have nasal resonance, they do not have audible nasal airflow. This latter is not normally encountered in natural language (although the voiceless nasals encountered in some languages may well have a certain degree of audible nasal escape), but is relatively frequent in patients with velopharyngeal insufficiency. It may occur both with target nasals (which may in this case be termed nareal fricatives) and accompanying other articulation types.

Finally in this section we consider velopharyngeal friction. This is the loud friction resulting from air leakage through a tense, but incompletely occluded, velopharyngeal port. This may occur by itself (the so-called "nasal-snort") or accompanying other articulations. For these two cases, a symbol and a diacritic to mark a particular aspect of nasal sound release not found in normal speech is required.

Segment Length

Length is often considered a prosodic aspect and as such is dealt with in more detail in Chapter 6. But we can mention here that consonants (as much as vowels—see later) can differ in length. In IPA practice consonant length is often marked by doubling the symbol, although the use of the length mark—[:]—can also be employed. It is normally assumed that two degrees of consonant length are all that need be marked for most languages. In disordered speech, however, clinical phoneticians may well need a greater degree of flexibility than that, as prolongation of segments is attested in several types of speech disorder, ranging from disfluency to acquired neurological disorders.

The IPA now provides three marks of length: one for an extra short sound: [ă], one for a half-long sound: [aˑ], and one for a long sound: [aː]; the unmarked symbol being interpreted as being of a "normal" length for the particular sound and language concerned. In transcribing disordered speech one can employ combinations of the half-long and long, and/or double use of the long marks to show prolonged articulation of varying lengths. Usually, the extra short diacritic is sufficient to mark sounds shorter than normal, as degrees of "shortness" are difficult to perceive, and it is therefore unlikely that a great deal of exactness will be required in their transcription.

Double and Secondary Articulations

As noted above, double articulations of varying types may occur in disordered speech, including some combinations (such as alveolar-velar stops) that are unusual in natural language. However, the IPA's tie-bar diacritic (e.g., [k͡p]) can be applied to any double articulations and these, therefore, do not present a problem to the transcriber.

Secondary articulations of various unusual types (such as labio-dental secondary articulation with lingual consonants) may also be transcribed relatively easily through extending the practice of superscript letters recommended by the IPA for such secondary features as labialization and palatalization. One feature not so easily dealt with is spread-lip shape (the opposite of labialized), for which no current IPA symbol seems to suffice, along with the difference between close and open-rounded labialization. Many of these secondary articulation features can be found also affecting entire stretches of speech. In such cases, we consider them aspects of the voice quality of the speaker and this area is returned to in detail in Chapter 6.

Plosives

Finally, we consider the adaptations that occur with plosives. These include nasal and lateral release, aspiration, and affrication. Although these are all quite normal in natural language (including English, in which examples of all of these features occur), one can encounter less typical examples for specific languages. For English, these might include lateral and nasal release from places of articulation other than alveolar and affricates other than palato-alveolar. All these can be shown quite adequately using current IPA conventions.

Vowels

Again using the check-list of articulatory parameters provided in Ball (1993), the following features can be examined.

Airstream Mechanism and Direction

Although not impossible, vowel-like sounds are only very rarely encountered on nonpulmonic airstreams (with the exception of esophageal/tracheo-esophageal and electrolarynx speech). Nevertheless, although we can be almost categorical about the airstream, it is quite possible to vary the direction. Just as it was seen with consonants that a pulmonic ingressive air flow could be used, so one can find the same with vowels. In other words, a pulmonic ingressive airstream can be used for whole stretches of speech, either pathologically or for some extra-linguistic purpose, such as to disguise the voice.

Phonation

It is often assumed that vowels are always voiced. However, voiceless vowels can be produced, and do occur in some languages (they are often heard, for example, in French). It might be claimed that a voiceless vowel is actually a type of fricative as, when they are used in natural language, there is generally an audible breathy quality to them: Without this, they would clearly be inaudible. This quality is brought about by a slight narrowing of the channel through which the air flows and so they may well resemble voiceless fricatives of varying types. Nevertheless, where the sound is substituted for a target voiced vowel in disordered speech, it is probably best to transcribe it with the vowel symbol and the IPA voiceless diacritic, as this explicitly shows the link between the target and the realization (e.g., [i̥]).

Tongue Height

Vowels are usually described in terms of the position of the highest point of the tongue arch on two axes: the vertical and the horizontal. In terms of the vertical axis, tongue height has normally been divided into four main categories: high (with the tongue closest to the palate), half-high, half-low, and low. Alternative labels are close, half-close, half-open, and open, which are standard in Europe. Indeed, the cardinal vowel system (see Ball, 1993, for a description of this system) has cardinal vowels at these four different tongue heights (although the claim is that in the cardinal vowel system, the vowels represent auditorily determined rather than articulatorily determined points).

This should not be construed, however, to mean that only four different degrees of height can be distinguished. By using the diacritics that are provided by the IPA, phoneticians can mark vowels that are higher or lower from the usual (or "cardinal") value of a particular symbol. This is not particularly precise, however. In other words, it would be difficult to distinguish between a vowel that was slightly higher than a particular value and another that was higher still but not yet high enough to be classed as "lower" than the next cardinal value. Normally, even in disordered speech, such a degree of precision is not required, and the set of diacritics provided is generally sufficient. Figures 2–2 and 2–3 in Chapter 2 show vowel symbols described in this section and the use of diacritics.

Frontness-Backness of the Tongue

Looking at the horizontal axis, one can see that the highest point on the tongue arch can adopt a variety of positions. In phonetics, generally three such positions are recognized: front, mid/central, and back. Again, the IPA (1993, its most recent revision) assigns vowel symbols to all three positions at all the heights except low. At the low position, the distance between the front and back vowels is smaller (because of the shape of the vowel area), but even here one can denote vowels in a mid position through the use of diacritics.

Vowels advanced somewhat from a back or central value can be shown with diacritics, as can vowels retracted somewhat from the front or central values. A diacritic also exists to mark a central vowel: this now is only of use for the fully low position (as previously noted) for the other heights now have assigned vowel symbols for the central position.

A recent innovation that links the vertical and horizontal axes is a diacritic to mark "mid-centralized," a vowel that is moved towards the absolute center of the vowel area. The use of this sign avoids the necessity to use two diacritics for this sort of vowel (e.g., a lowering and retraction mark or a raising and advanced mark). Figure 2–3 shows the use of diacritics on a vowel diagram to chart vowel values.

In some languages, vowels differ not only in the two axes discussed, but also in the position of the tongue root. Two different vowels may have identical tongue body position, but the tongue root may be retracted into the pharynx for one and in an advanced position for the other. The IPA now provides diacritics for these differences, which might on occasion be useful for clinical transcription.

Lip Shape

The third main vowel parameter is lip shape. Often, the only two values listed here are rounded versus unrounded, as such a two-way distinction appears to be the maximum utilized phonologically in natural language. Nevertheless, phoneticians often use a three-way distinction between rounded, neutral, and spread. For vowels, certain symbols stand for rounded vowels and certain for spread vowels, with a vowel such as the mid-central schwa ([ə]) assumed to have neutral lip shape.

For consonants, the IPA currently provides a diacritic to mark labialization (i.e., lip-rounding), but does not sanction any sign to mark lip-spreading. For the transcription of speech disorders, we can imagine that it may well be important to have a sign to mark that a spread-lip shape was used when one might have expected a neutral or rounded shape.

With vowels, it is also worth noting that the high rounded vowels have a tighter degree of rounding than do lower ones and likewise for the spread lip vowels: the higher they are, the more spread is the lip shape. The IPA currently has diacritics to mark when these expectations are not met for rounded vowels: to show a lip shape more round than expected and less round than expected. This does not extend to spread vowels however.

Secondary Articulation

The only secondary articulation that is normally described for vowels is retroflexion or rhoticization. Vowels can be pronounced with the tip of the tongue curled back to a greater or lesser extent, and this is often how postvocalic "r" is pronounced in rhotic accents of English. The IPA provides a diacritic to mark this tongue shape.

The full list of IPA vowel diacritics just discussed is as follows:

advanced	[a̟]	retracted	[a̠]
raised	[a̝]	lowered	[ɛ̞]
advanced tongue root	[a̘]	retracted tongue root	[a̙]
mid-centralized	[ě]	rhoticized	[ɚ]
more rounded	[ɔ̹]	less rounded	[ɔ̜]

Amount of Tongue Tension

As with the force of articulation parameter with consonants, vowels can be classed as tense or lax, depending on the amount of tongue tension used in their production. Tense vowels tend to be nearer the periphery of the vowel area (and often longer and louder), with lax vowels tending to be more centralized (and often shorter and quieter). The IPA provides a series of "spare" vowel symbols that are often used to denote lax vowels in particular languages. For example, in transcribing English (with most accents having several such lax vowels), one often uses the following spare symbols /ɪ, æ, ʊ/. The mid-central vowel (or "schwa") is often thought of as a lax vowel and is symbolized as /ə/: this vowel is very common in unstressed syllables in English.

No diacritics exist to distinguish tense from lax vowels, but the use of the spare symbols or the use of diacritics to mark nonperipheral status is usually sufficient to mark vowels as lax. Diacritics designed to show strong or weak articulation (see under Consonants) could be utilized, particularly if there is a need to note vowels that are particularly loud or quiet.

Length of Vowel

As with consonants, vowels are measurable in time and can be classed as short, "normal," half-long, and long. The latest version of the IPA provides diacritics for shorter and longer vowels than normal for the vowel and language under study; the absence of such diacritics can be read as meaning the normal length. They can be illustrated as follows:

shorter than normal	[ă]
normal	[ɑ]
half-long	[ɑˑ]
long	[ɑː]

There are no guidelines for what distinguishes half-long from fully long, but it is assumed that this corresponds to perceivable rather than measurable differences.

As we stated with consonant length, longer vowels that might occur in disordered speech can be marked by repeated use of the half-long and long diacritics.

Vowel Stability

Under this heading we can consider diphthongs. Vocalic elements containing a marked difference in quality (i.e., tongue position) between the onset and the end and that constitute a single syllable only are termed diphthongs. Diphthongs are normally transcribed with two vowel symbols: one to represent the quality of the initial and the other the final part of the sound. Usually this is sufficient; however, should it be necessary to distinguish diphthongs from two abutting monophthongs (i.e., two neighboring vowels belonging to separate syllables), one can use the IPA linking diacritic to mark the diphthong, and the syllable break mark to show abutting monophthongs:

diphthong	[a͜i]
two monophthongs	[a.i]

The practice sometimes encountered of marking diphthongs by placing a long straight line (a macron) over the two vowels is not recognized by the IPA, and is potentially confusing, as some systems use macrons to mark length. It should thus be avoided.

Nasality/Orality

Nasal vowels occur frequently in natural language, both as phonemes (e.g., French) or as allophones of otherwise oral vowels (e.g., English). These nasal vowels can be shown by the use of the tilde diacritic: [ã]. Vowels following nasal consonants will often be partially (rather than fully) nasalized at the beginning of the vowel, and vowels preceding nasal consonants will often be partially nasalized at the end of the vowel. The IPA does not provide any means of marking such partially nasalized vowels, but there could be circumstances—in the transcription of disordered speech—for which it might be felt useful to have this ability. We return to this problem later.

Finally, the features of nasal friction and velopharyngeal friction noted under Consonants can also occur with vowels and have no accepted IPA symbolization.

Prosodic Features

As we have mentioned before, prosodic aspects of transcription are mentioned in greater detail in Chapters 6 and 7. However, we will introduce some of the issues here to illustrate the range of prosodic features that may occur in disordered speech.

By definition, prosodic features are phonetic features that spread over more than one segment. However, the domain of different features may differ considerably. For example, an intonation "tune" may operate over a single syllable (such as "yes?") or over several words (e.g., "thank-you very much indeed"). Features such as stress operate over single syllables, although voice quality may be constant over the entire utterances of a speaker.

A great need in transcription, therefore, is the ability to notate which portion of the transcription the particular prosodic feature applies to. However, apart from the provision of some diacritics to mark stress and tone, the IPA does not have a wide range of symbolization for prosodic features.

Some of the features that can be characterized as prosodic (or suprasegmental) and that may need to be characterized in a clinical transcription if disordered are now covered further.

Stress and Rhythm

Here is needed the ability to transcribe not only stress placement (where unusual placement will clearly affect rhythm), but also excessively heavy or light stress. Fortunately, this is relatively straightforward through the use of the IPA-sanctioned stress marks.

Pitch and Intonation

There are a large number of methods of transcribing the use of pitch in intonation, as discussed in Chapter 6, and the IPA does not sanction any particular system. The sorts of problems encountered in dysprosody (as described in Chapter 7) are however normally easily notated by most of these systems.

Phonatory and Supraglottal Aspects of Voice Quality

Although much work has been undertaken (see Laver, 1980) on describing aspects of voice quality derived from both phonatory activity and supraglottal articulatory settings, there has not been an agreed set of symbols for transcribing these. The IPA has a few diacritics for marking individual symbols with particular phonation types (voiced, voiceless, breathy voiced, creaky voiced), but no method of marking stretches of speech uttered with a particular voice quality. It also lacks symbols for other phonatory types such as whisper and falsetto, which are often encountered in the clinic. It has no symbols for supraglottal voice qualities. Fortunately recent work in this area (see Ball, Esling, & Dickson, in press) has attempted to fill this gap, and is reported on in Chapter 6.

Pausing

The use of pauses is common in both normal and disordered speech. Despite this, the IPA has no means to mark pauses. As shown in Chapter 6, various methods have been proposed by researchers into conversational analysis. What is needed is a clear and unambiguous method of marking pauses of varying lengths, so that a transcription can clearly indicate whether the use of pauses is within normal bounds or not.

Tempo and Loudness

Again, there is no way within the IPA and most other transcription conventions for marking speed of speech and loudness. Clearly, with some patient types (such as those with hearing impairment) such information may be important. Researchers into conversation analysis often note such information, sometimes through the adaptation of musical notation. Such a conclusion is illustrated in Chapter 6.

All of these are dealt with in some detail in Chapter 6, where the novel method of marking the domain of the feature devised by clinical phoneticians will be introduced.

Principles for Symbolizing Disordered Speech

If new symbols for the transcription of atypical speech are to be created, there are several principles to bear in mind.

1. Compatibility. The IPA is the most widely known, used, and accepted system of phonetic transcription in the world, and so in devising new symbols, one should take care that they are compatible with the IPA. By that we mean that symbols used in any new system should not already be used by the IPA or be confusable with those of the IPA. Notions such as placement of diacritics for secondary articulations and so on should be kept the same as far as possible and the general appearance of symbol shapes should not jar with those of the IPA. It is probable that for most occasions, symbols for atypical pronunciations will be mixed with those for normal speech (i.e., the IPA), so it helps if they blend in well.

2. Comprehensiveness. We do not want ad hoc design of new symbols off-the-cuff, where one clinical phonetician will not understand the symbols of another. Therefore, a comprehensive design process is sought, where the atypical pronunciations we need to cover are identified (as done here), and a set of symbols for these behaviors is discussed and agreed upon by as wide a range of practitioners as possible, and then publicized to other clinicians.

3. Frequency of occurrence. However, it is desirable to avoid the temptation to create vast numbers of symbols to cover every possible disordered pronunciation however rarely it occurs. It is necessary to distinguish, therefore, between rare behaviors that can be described quite easily in a footnote and those that occur sufficiently often that an agreed symbolization will make the clinical transcriber's life easier.

4. Symbols and Diacritics. A distinction can be drawn between an entire symbol and a diacritical mark to be added to a symbol. Often, the atypical behaviors clinical phoneticians are trying to describe involve some kind of adaptation to a normal behavior: in which case a diacritic can be added to an existing IPA symbol to show this change. On other occasions, clinical phoneticians are looking at ways to describe something totally different from normal speech: Here a new symbol is more warranted. Let us give an example. If dentolabial articulation is found, one can clearly see its relation to labiodental. In this case, therefore, a diacritic can be designed that would apply to symbols for labial consonants to show that the precise type of labial constriction in this case was upper lip to lower teeth. However, one may also encounter a sound made by banging the upper and lower teeth together, and this bidental percussive would be unlike any other normal sound and so would require a new symbol to transcribe it.

In the last 15 years or so, there have been several attempts to extend the set of symbols and diacritics to account for aspects of disordered speech. Unfortunately, most of these have failed to meet one or more of the principles we have just described. They mainly lacked comprehensibility (by focusing on one particular area). Also, not being sponsored by any particular organization, one finds competing symbols for the same features among the schemes.

Among those attempts were those by Bush et al. (1973, cited in Ingram 1976), who concentrated on consonants in child language; Dalton & Hardcastle (1977), whose main interest was in transcribing disfluent speech; and Laver (1980), whose focus was voice quality. Shriberg and Kent (1982) had a broader approach and many of their symbols have become known quite widely in the U.S. Vieregge (1987) also drew up a fairly wide set of symbols and his work has been known mostly in Europe. Vieregge's system is notable for its inclusion of a sophisticated means of marking how certain one is of the accuracy of a particular symbol.

A major attempt to expand symbolization was made by a group of British phoneticians and speech pathologists through the early 1980s. This group—the Phonetic Representation of Disordered Speech group (PRDS)—was first convened in 1979, publishing a preliminary report after a year (PRDS, 1980), with a final report later (1983). Many of the problems outlined here were covered by this group, which kept fairly close to the principles we have just outlined. Little published work used the symbols (see Ball, 1988, for more details), and before they could become more widely known, they were overtaken by the developments at the 1989 Convention of the IPA held in Kiel, Germany.

That convention established a working group to examine the symbolization of disordered speech and of normal and disordered voice quality. Many of the suggestions of PRDS and of scholars such as Shriberg and Kent and of Vieregge were accepted, but changes were also needed, as some of the symbols suggested by PRDS, for example, had been adopted at Kiel by the IPA to stand for other sounds. The set of symbols prepared by this working group was termed "The Extensions to the IPA for the transcription of disordered speech and voice quality," and has become known as extIPA ([ɛkˈstaɪpə]) for short, and is described in full in Duckworth, Allen, Hardcastle, and Ball (1990). Since the Kiel Congress, several additions have been made to the set and the current version is given in Figure 4–1 and in the Appendix. A fuller set of symbols for voice quality than is provided in extIPA has recently been established (see Ball, Esling, & Dickson, in press), termed VoQS (Voice Quality Symbols) and this is described in Chapter 6.

ExtIPA Proposals for Clinical Transcription

As has just been discussed, the Extensions to the IPA (extIPA) were devised in 1989, being revised slightly since, as noted in Ball (1993) and Bernhardt and Ball (1993). These proposals go a long way to meeting the requirements noted in the previous sections on consonants and vowels, as well as dealing with some of the

CONSONANTS (other than those on the IPA Chart)

	bilabial	labiodental	dentolabial	labioalv.	linguolabial	interdental	bidental	alveolar	velar	velophar.
Plosive	p̪ b̪		p͆ b͆	p̺ b̺	t̼ d̼	t̪ d̪				
Nasal			m͆	m̺	n̼	n̪				
Trill					r̼	r̪				
Fricative median			f͆ v͆	f̺ v̺	θ̼ ð̼	θ̪ ð̪	ħ̪ ɦ̪			ꞯ
Fricative lateral+ median								ʪ ʫ		
Fricative nareal	m̃							ñ	ŋ̃	
Percussive	w̥ w̥						ŋ̩			
Approximant lateral					l̼	l̪				

DIACRITICS

↔ labial spreading	s̞	‖ strong articulation	f̬	~ denasal	m̃
͆ dentolabial	v̪	ꟷ weak articulation	v̥	÷ nasal escape	ṽ̇
̼ interdental/bidental	n̼	\ reiterated articulation	p\p\p	꞊ velopharyngeal friction	s̄
= alveolar	t̠	→ whistled articulation	s̝	↓ ingressive airflow	p↓
‿ linguolabial	d̼	→ sliding articulation	θs̠	↑ egressive airflow	!↑

CONNECTED SPEECH

(.)	short pause
(..)	medium pause
(...)	long pause
f	loud speech [{f laʊd f}]
ff	louder speech [{ff laʊdə ff}]
p	quiet speech [{p kwaɪət p}]
pp	quieter speech [{pp kwaɪətə pp}]
allegro	fast speech [{allegro faːst allegro}]
lento	slow speech [{ lento sloʊ lento}]
crescendo, ralentando, etc may also be used

VOICING

˰	pre-voicing	˰z
˯	post-voicing	z˯
(ͺ)	partial devoicing	(z̥)
(ͺ	initial partial devoicing	(z̥
ͺ)	final partial devoicing	z̥)
(ͺ)	partial voicing	(s̬)
(ͺ	initial partial voicing	(s̬
ͺ)	final partial voicing	s̬)
=	unaspirated	p=
h	pre-aspiration	ʰp

OTHERS

(◌̲)	indeterminate sound	() silent articulation	(ʃ)
(V̲)	indeterminate vowel	(()) extraneous noise	((2 sylls))
(Pl̲)	indeterminate plosive	* sound with no symbol available	
(Pl,vls)	indeterminate voiceless plosive, etc	(to be described elsewhere)	

Figure 4–1. extIPA Chart 1994. (Reprinted with permission.)

requirements for suprasegementals. Here, we will deal only with the symbolization for consonants and vowels; prosodic aspects are dealt with in Chapters 6 and 7.

Consonants

Only those subsections (or parts of them) are included below where the IPA does not have sufficient symbols to deal with the atypical speech features identified previously.

Airstream Mechanism and Direction

To mark pulmonic ingressive speech, extIPA provides a downward pointing arrow that may be placed after the symbol for the sound that was pronounced ingressively, for example [p↓]. Should it be necessary to mark egressive velaric sounds (i.e., reverse clicks), one can employ an upward pointing arrow—[!↑]—although such sounds are not particularly common. The arrows by themselves can be used to mark inhalation and exhalation should that be necessary.[1]

If one wishes to mark that a stretch of speech was uttered on a pulmonic ingressive airstream rather than a single segment, then one can use the extIPA innovation of the labeled braces. The stretch of speech affected is enclosed within brace brackets that are marked with the downward arrow (or whatever other feature one wishes to note taking place across the stretch). We illustrate this by showing the effect of counting using alternatively egressive and ingressive air:

['wʌn {↓ 'tuː ↓} 'θɹiː {↓'fɔːɹ ↓}]—"one, two, three, four"

Similarly, esophageal speech will need to be marked over an utterance rather than on single segments. The labeled brace approach can also be used here, although the suggested symbol naturally differs. Here we use [Œ], to stand for the original Latin spelling of oesophagus. An example is given as follows:

[{Œ 'haʊ ɑːɹ 'juː Œ}]—"how are you?"

Phonation

Fine distinctions within the voiced-voiceless contrast can be marked under the extIPA conventions. Through the use of brackets around the diacritics used for

---

[1]The arrows used for ingressive and egressive airflow are potentially confusable with IPA symbols for upstep and downstep in intonation. These latter, however, are shorter than the extIPA symbols [↑], [↓] as compared to extIPA [↑], [↓].

voiced and voiceless, one can show partial voicing of a normally voiceless consonant and partial devoicing of a normally voiced consonant as in [z] and [f]. If one wishes to show that this partial devoicing or partial voicing was at the initial part of the segment in question, one uses only a left parenthesis, if one wishes to show that it was at the final part of the segment, one uses the diacritic with only the right parenthesis. These are shown in:

partial voicing (initial)	[ˌs̬]
partial voicing (final)	[s̬ˌ]
partial devoicing (initial)	[ˌz̥]
partial devoicing (final)	[z̥ˌ]

Finally, we may wish to show that voicing for a particular voiced segment started early and/or continued beyond the end of the segment where the context (such as utterance final) would have expected it to have stopped. One can show this quite clearly by placing the voice diacritic (with no parentheses) to the left or right of the relevant symbol: [ˌz] and [zˌ].

Preaspiration was also noted in the previous discussion. As normal aspiration is noted by a superscript-h after the symbol ([pʰ]), extIPA simply extends this usage to before the symbol to show preaspiration: [ʰp].

Strength of Articulation

ExtIPA symbols for extra strong and extra weak articulation are as follows:

[f̎]	extra strong
[m̮]	extra weak

These could also be used in transcribing normal speech to mark fortis and lenis consonants, should this be desired.

Place of Articulation

A number of new symbols and diacritics are provided by extIPA for atypical places of articulation and, indeed, a few of the innovations in the 1989 IPA chart are useful for the clinical phonetician, as well. The following are the means of transcribing the various places noted above, shown with typical symbols:

linguo-labials	t̼
labio-dentals	p̪ b̪
dento-labials	p̃

labio-alveolars	m̲
interdentals	n̪
bidental approximation	ʊ̪
bidental percussive	n̥
bilabial percussive	w̥
alveolar diacritic	d̲
pharyngeal plosives	ʠ ɢ
sliding articulation	ʃ↘s

Manner of Articulation

The manner types discussed above can be transcribed in the following way:

reiteration	[pʰ/pʰ/pʰ], [sə/sə/sə]
whistled articulation	[↑S]

Central Versus Lateral Articulation

ExtIPA provides two symbols to cover fricatives that have both a central and lateral release. Adapting the model of the symbol for the voiced alveolar lateral fricative, which is a combination of a lateral symbol and a fricative symbol, these combine aspects of the symbols for alveolar central and lateral fricatives. They are [ʪ] for the voiceless one, and [ʫ] for the voiced.

Nasality/Orality

The various categories of nasality and orality discussed previously can be represented by the following symbols and diacritics:

denasal	m̄
nasal escape	v̈
nareal fricatives	m̈ n̈ ŋ̈ etc.
velopharyngeal friction	s̃
velopharyngeal fricative	fŋ

Length

As previously stated, the current set of length marks can be used to notate atypical length of segments quite easily. For example, [ɑː] might be used for a vowel slightly longer than normal, while [ɑːː] or [ɑːːː] would show excessive length. Very short segments can be shown as [m̆].

Secondary Articulations

To show close rounding and open rounding as secondary articulations, we can use the diacritics proposed in the VoQS system. This uses the IPA labialization diacritic for close rounding (e.g., [tʷ]) and for open rounding uses a superscript cardinal vowel 11: [tꟳ]. Spread lip shape is shown through the use of a new diacritic in extIPA: the double-headed arrow placed beneath the symbol, as in [ꭍ↔].

Vowels

Again, we include only those subsections for which the IPA does not have adequate symbols, with the discussion in the preceding section providing answers to some of the queries raised for vowels in atypical speech.

Airstream Direction

As with consonants we can use the downward pointing arrow to mark ingressive vowels.

Phonation

Voiceless vowels can be marked as [i̥, ẙ, u̥]. However, as noted above, they have a fricative quality, so an alternative transcription could be as follows: [ⁱç, ʸçʷ, ᵘxʷ], with the raised vowel symbols marking the short amount of voiced vowel that normally occurs at the beginning. For the two rounded examples we have included the labialization diacritic.

Lip-Spread Vowels

One can note lip-spread vowels with the double-headed arrow diacritic already discussed for consonants.

Orality/Nasality

Apart from the discussion of denasalization, nasal friction and velopharyngeal friction covered above under consonants, we might wish to consider how to denote degrees of nasalization. As we saw with voicing, extIPA sanction the use of diacritics to mark partial voicing/devoicing at initial or final position within a segment. Although there are no specific proposals in extIPA, it would seem we could adapt the same procedure to mark nasalization being particularly strong at the beginning or end of a vowel by offsetting the tilde diacritic to the left or to the right; e.g.: [˜ɑ] or [ɑ˜]. It is unlikely, however, that such a degree of accuracy will be needed often.

In this chapter we have explored aspects of atypical speech that may need to be transcribed by the speech-language pathologist, and have provided the most current and widely accepted set of symbols to deal with them. In the following chapter we will explore the use of phonetic transcription within the clinical context in more detail.

CHAPTER

⑤

The Clinical Use of Phonetic Transcription

In this chapter we look at how phonetic transcription is used in the clinical situation as a tool to aid in the analysis (and therefore the effective treatment) of speech disorders. In the first part of the chapter we will examine the amount of detail required in clinical transcription, following that with a discussion of whether transcription can aid in making distinctions between types of speech disorder (phonetic versus phonological). We conclude by examining some examples of the use of the symbols described in the previous chapter.

Broad and Narrow Transcription

Approaches to the task of phonetic transcription as noted in Chapter 2 reflect different approaches to describing speech in general. Phoneticians are interested in the speech production and reception mechanisms and the acoustic signal of speech and describe these features as accurately as possible without regard to the role the sounds, themselves, play in language. Linguists—or more precisely—phonologists are, however, concerned mainly in the patterns of sound within language rather than the minutiae of the sounds, themselves. This results in two different transcription traditions: that which tries to capture as much phonetic detail as possible, and that which only wishes to identify linguistically meaningful units. As noted in Chapter 2, these two approaches have been termed "phonetic" and "phonemic/phonological" and "narrow" and "broad."

However, these two pairs of labels are not totally interchangeable and are not always used in a precise way. The distinction between "phonetic" and "phonemic" should be clear: a phonetic transcription in this sense attempts to capture enough detail to mark the distinctive allophones of the phonemes of a language (so perhaps the term "allophonic" is better here, so we can keep "phonetic" as a general umbrella term for any kind of transcription), with "phonemic" providing only one symbol per phoneme, ignoring allophonic variation. Clearly, a phonemic transcription can only be read accurately by someone who is already acquainted with the phonology of the language and, as such, is not suitable for the purposes of illustrating a language's pronunciation to those who have no prior knowledge of the language.

"Narrow" and "broad" transcriptions as terms are, however, not necessarily tied to the notions of allophone and phoneme. They imply simply a difference between a detailed and a simple transcription. Although an allophonic transcription will tend to be detailed (and so "narrow"), the degree of detail will depend on whether only main allophones or all perceptible differences are being recorded. Likewise, although a phonemic transcription is bound to be broad, we may also get fairly simple transcriptions that contain some allophonic (and so not strictly "phonemic") information.

The difference between these two terms is relevant for the use of phonetic transcription of disordered speech in the clinic. Clearly, a patient presenting with disordered speech will be demonstrating some degree of disruption (whether mild or severe) of the phonological patterns of their native accent. As the phonology is disrupted, one cannot use a phonemic transcription, as that usage assumes a normal phonology. We must, therefore, adopt an approach that does not record phonemic units, but attempts to describe phonetic features.

We turn, therefore, to the simple distinction in terms of amount of detail: "broad" versus "narrow." As with many clinical procedures confronting the speech-language pathologist, there is a tension here between speed and depth. It is naturally less time-consuming to undertake a transcription that involves marking the least amount of detail possible, however the price paid for this is lack of depth in the analysis. If such lack of depth still allowed adequate classifications of errors, this would not be a problem and broad transcriptions would be perfectly acceptable; however, as we will seek to demonstrate, lack of detail may well result in misleading analyses.

There is, however, a further consideration. Although narrow transcriptions may well result in better analyses of disordered speech, the more detail that is required of a transcriber, the greater the room for transcription error and uncertainty. This point is also detailed in the following section.

We now look at some examples of clinical transcription in which the difference between a broad and narrow approach can be vital in arriving at a correct analysis (and, therefore, treatment) of the disordered phonology of the patient.

The following sample is given first in broad transcription; as all these transcriptions are nonphonemic (for reasons previously noted), square brackets are used throughout and we note which are broad and which narrow (although this is, to some extent, obvious from the amount of detail included).

Speaker A. Age 7;3. Broad Transcription.

shop	[ʃɑːp]	shoe	[ʃuː]
see	[ʃiː]	seat	[ʃiːt]
ship	[ʃɪp]	wash	[wɑːʃ]
sip	[ʃɪp]	yes	[jeʃ]
rush	[ɹʌʃ]	kiss	[kɪʃ]
cushion	[ˈkʊʃən]	messy	[ˈmeʃi]

This sample appears to be a clear example of the loss of phonological contrast between two target phonemes of English: /s/ and /ʃ/, with [ʃ] being used for both in all places of word structure. Indeed, the minimal pair "sip" and "ship" are in the sample and appear to show a homonymic clash in speaker A's speech. However, this is a broad transcription, in which the transcriber has restricted the symbol set to those normally encountered in the transcription of adult target English phonology. In examining a narrower transcription of the same data, in which other IPA symbols are utilized, a different picture emerges:

Speaker A. Age 7;3. Narrow Transcription.

shop	[ʃɑːp]	shoe	[ʃuː]
see	[çiː]	seat	[çiːt]
ship	[ʃɪp]	wash	[wɑːʃ]
sip	[çɪp]	yes	[jeç]
rush	[ɹʌʃ]	kiss	[kɪç]
cushion	[ˈkʊʃən]	messy	[ˈmeçi]

On examination of this transcription, it is seen that actually this speaker has *not* lost the contrast between target /s/ and /ʃ/. It is true that they are not realized in the standard way, but although [ç] is not a phoneme of English and will sound extremely odd being used for /s/, homonymic clashes do not result from this pronunciation and so the contrast between words will not be lost.

The treatment approach for a patient lacking a phonological contrast will naturally differ from that needed for a patient whose phonology is intact, but whose phonetic realization of some phonemes is disordered. The clinician working from the broad transcription may schedule needless time attempting to establish contrasts through minimal pair practice, when what is actually required is work on the realization of /s/ alone.

This first example involves a major simplification of the transcription process in the broad version, in that the difference between a post-alveolar and a palatal fricative should be quite noticeable and is lost in the transcription simply because the transcriber chose only the English consonant set. We can demonstrate other examples in which the phonetic difference is not so great, but the importance of narrow transcription is equally clear.

Speaker B. Age 6;9. Broad Transcription.

pin	[pɪn]	ten	[ten]
bin	[pɪn]	den	[ten]
cot	[kɑːt]	pea	[piː]
got	[kɑːt]	bee	[piː]

This data set also suggests that there is a collapse of phonological contrast: specifically the contrast between voiced and voiceless plosives in word-initial position. This clearly leads to homonymic clashes between, for example, "pin" and "bin" and "cot" and "got," respectively. As word-initial plosives have a high functional load in English, such a loss of the feature contrast [±voice] in this context clearly requires treatment. It would appear from this data, that an initial stage of treatment would concentrate on the establishment of the notion of contrast with this sound, before going on to practice the phonetic realization of this contrast.

However, if we look at a narrow transcription of the same data, the picture alters.

Speaker B. Age 6;9. Narrow Transcription.

pin	[pʰɪn]	ten	[tʰen]
bin	[pɪn]	den	[ten]
cot	[kʰɑːt]	pea	[pʰiː]
got	[kɑːt]	bee	[piː]

Again, it is clear from this transcription that there is not, actually, a loss of contrast between initial voiced and voiceless plosives. Target voiceless plosives are realized without vocal fold vibration (voice), but with aspiration on release (as are the adult target forms). The target voiced plosives are realized without aspiration (as with the adult forms), but also without any vocal fold vibration. It is this last difference that distinguishes them from the target form. For, although adult English "voiced" plosives are often devoiced for some of their duration in initial position, totally voiceless examples are rare.

The narrow transcription shows, therefore, that the difference between the speaker's pronunciation of these sounds and the target is minimal. The notion of contrast does not need to be established, and, as aspiration is the main acoustic cue used by adults to perceive the difference between these groups of plosives, the child's speech may well sound only slightly atypical.

We examine one more example in which the choice of transcription suggests a more limited phonology than is the case. Here the focus is on structural rather than systemic aspects of the speaker's phonology.

Speaker C. Age 6;10. Broad Transcription.

snow	[hnoʊ]	smile	[hmaɪl]
snake	[hneɪk]	smoke	[hmoʊk]
slow	[ɬoʊ]	swim	[hwɪm]
slide	[ɬaɪd]	sweet	[hwiːt]

This transcription presents a confusing picture of the target /s/+sonorant clusters. It appears that in all but "sl" clusters, the cluster is retained with a change of target /s/ to [h] (a change, incidentally quite common in historical phonology). In "sl" clusters there appears to be a replacement of both the /s/ and the /l/ by [ɬ]. This last might be thought of as an example of cluster reduction, although it is unclear if there is deletion of /s/ and substitution of /l/, or deletion of /l/ and substitution of /s/. This problem is clarified on examination of a narrow transcription of the same sample:

Speaker C. Age 6;10. Narrow Transcription.

snow	[n̥oʊ]	smile	[m̥aɪl]
snake	[n̥eɪk]	smoke	[m̥oʊk]
slow	[ɬoʊ]	swim	[ʍɪm]
slide	[ɬaɪd]	sweet	[ʍiːt]

This transcription illustrates that the use of [h] in the broad transcription was an attempt to capture the voiceless nature of the sonorants. The added friction with the realization of "sl" clusters prompted the use of the symbol for the voiceless lateral fricative, but in the other instances, the audible voiceless breath flow was interpreted as an added /h/. This transcription also shows that the speaker was not in fact using two different strategies with these clusters and there was no /s/ → [h] change involved. In all instances, there is reduction of a two-member cluster to a single sound. This sound, however, is not one of the two target sounds, but contains features from both target sounds. This process is often termed "feature synthesis," and it can be seen that what is retained in this sample is the place and manner of the second segment (e.g. alveolar and nasal, alveolar and lateral) with the voicelessness and friction of the first segment. This results in all the subject's initial segments in this sample being voiceless and to a lesser or greater degree fricative (e.g. with considerable friction in [ɬ] and [ʍ], and audible breath with the nasals).

This subject, then, has actually not mastered consonant clusters (at least with these target cluster types), but has clearly attempted to produce features associated with both sounds in the target cluster. In normal phonological development, feature synthesis is often found just prior to the acquisition of clusters, so this would suggest an intervention strategy related to the expansion of these initial sounds into full clusters. Working from the broad transcription, however, a change from [h] to /s/ is indicated, with the "sl" clusters as a separate problem: In other words, the generalization that unites these pronunciations into a single phonological process is lost.

The samples examined so far have all shown the broad transcription underestimating the ability of the patient. There can be, albeit less often, also instances in which broad transcriptions may overestimate the phonological development of the patient. This may occur when the transcriber self-limits to the symbols used in a phonemic transcription of English, or in which one allows influence by an expected sound (or both).

Speaker D. Age 7;2. Broad Transcription.

mat	[mæt͡s]	pat	[pæt͡s]
top	[t͡sɑːp]	tin	[t͡sɪn]
match	[mæt͡ʃ]	patch	[pæt͡ʃ]
chop	[t͡ʃɑːp]	chin	[t͡ʃɪn]

This transcription suggests that the speaker maintains a contrast between target /t/ and /tʃ/. The affricate appears to be pronounced as the adult target, with the plosive realized as an affricate at the alveolar place of articulation. However, in examining the narrow transcription, one can see that, in this instance, a restriction to the symbols used in transcribing adult English have led to an overestimation of this patient's abilities:

Speaker D. Age 7;2. Narrow Transcription.

mat	[mæt͡ʂ]	pat	[pæt͡ʂ]
top	[t͡ʂɑːp]	tin	[t͡ʂɪn]
match	[mæt͡ʂ]	patch	[pæt͡ʂ]
chop	[t͡ʂɑːp]	chin	[t͡ʂɪn]

This speaker uses a retroflex affricate for both target /t/ and /tʃ/. The expected alveolar and post-alveolar positions appear to have influenced the choice of symbols in the first transcription. The more detailed second transcription actually demonstrates that the contrast between these phonemes is lost and will need to be reestablished in therapy.

Further examples of how broad transcriptions can provide misleading data are given in Carney (1979). As mentioned here, however, there is also a price to pay for narrow transcription. One point often raised is that narrow transcription takes more time. This point is often posed in connection with detailed linguistic and phonetic analyses of disordered speech. Its validity as a criticism is suspect. Time spent on good analysis will save time wasted on ill-conceived and unjustified treatment. The real problem with this narrow phonetic approach lies with reliability. As noted in previous chapters, impressionistic transcription is essentially subjective, and its objectivity can only be tested through measuring how much agreement there is between different transcribers working to the same degree of detail and between transcriptions made by the same transcriber on different occasions. These reliability measures are termed inter- and intrascorer reliability, respectively. Studies have shown (e.g., Shriberg & Lof, 1991) that the narrower the transcription, the less reliable it is on both measures.

One of the reasons why narrow transcription of disordered (as opposed to normal) speech may lack reliability is, of course, that until recently many of the speech behaviors encountered in this type of speech had no recognized symbolization. It is to be hoped that the introduction of extIPA symbols (see Chapter 4), together with the development of new technology to aid the transcription process (see Chapter 9) will go some way to improve this situation. The main difficulty, however, is probably the lack of narrow phonetic training (see Chapter 3) in many training institutions. Such training has been a tradition in some areas (especially in Europe), but far too often transcription practice is restricted to phonemic approaches. Clearly, the ability to transcribe a normal phonemic system is of limited use to clinicians who encounter only speakers who do not use such a normal system!

Phonetic and Phonological Disorders

A common distinction between different types of speech disorders is that made between phonetic and phonological. This classification is based on the output of the disordered speech (rather than the input: see Code & Ball, 1988 and following), and so it might be thought that a transcription of a patient's speech output might be an aid to assigning a disorder to one type or the other.

A phonetic disorder is one in which target sounds are replaced by sounds that are not part of the phonemic inventory of the language (in that they are totally different), or they are phonetically similar, but perhaps the wrong allophone for the context. A phonological disorder is one in which the errors noted do involve the use of the wrong phoneme in the wrong place.

It would appear that a distinction such as the above could be easily captured through phonetic transcription. Indeed, the difference between these two bears a resemblance to the distinction between different degrees of transcription discussed in the previous chapter. In other words, a phonemic transcription or a broad phonetic transcription should be all that is needed to capture a speech disorder in which phonemic substitution or omission is all that is wrong. However, a narrow phonetic transcription would be required if the disordered speech involved sub-phonemic distortions or the use of nonnative phones. Of course, until one carries out a narrow transcription, one cannot usually tell whether a disorder is purely phonological or not.

Working on this hypothesis, therefore, one might think that a straightforward method of assigning speech data to the phonological or phonetic error categories would be to assess the transcription, and check it for the presence or otherwise of allophonic errors or sounds not normally encountered in the target language. However, there are several problems with the whole idea of a binary division of disordered speech. First, many speakers may well demonstrate a mixed-error type. By this we mean that they may have some phonemic errors as well as some phonetic errors. We demonstrate this with the following examples.

Speaker E.

ring	[ɹɪn]	key	[tiː]
rock	[ɹɑːt]	get	[det]
log	[lɒːd]	singing	[tɪnɪn]

Speaker F.

spin	[spʰɪn]	stamp	[stʰæmpˀ]
spider	[spʰaɪdɚ]	steady	[stʰedi]
scorn	[skʰɔːɹn]	skin	[skʰɪn]

With Speaker E, it is clear from the transcription that the disorder is one of substituting one phoneme for another, in this case alveolar sounds for corresponding velar ones (and also one /s/ ➝ /t/ substitution): this is an example of a phonological disorder type. With Speaker F, on the other hand, all the changes involve subphonemic distortions in that the aspirated, instead of the unaspirated, allophones of the fortis plosives are used following /s/ and so fits into the phonetic disorder type. However, let us look at something a little more complex:

Speaker G.

shop	[cɑːp]	shoe	[cuː]
soft	[ɬɒːft]	sell	[ɬel]
think	[fɪŋk]	thumb	[fʌm]
fat	[fæt]	fame	[feɪm]

This speaker clearly exhibits a mixed type of disorder. Some aspects are phonological: the substitution of the labio-dental fricatives for the dental in "think" and "thumb" involves the use of one phoneme of the target system for another. However, the use of the lateral fricative for target /s/ involves the use of a sound from outside the system of the target language and so cannot be phonological. Finally, the use of an alveo-palatal fricative for a target palato-alveolar fricative can be viewed either as a slight subphonemic distortion or as the use of a nonnative sound. But, whichever view is taken, it is still a phonetic rather than phonological feature.

This last point illustrates another problem with the distinction between phonetic and phonological disorders. Phonetic problems are counted as both sounds that are slightly different from those expected, and those that are very different, but from outside the system—and, what is more, it is not always easy to tell these varieties apart. Some authors only count allophonic differences as truly phonetic disorders; with these authors, however, it is not always easy to know what (if anything) one is supposed to do with any nonnative sounds.

Even if some of these difficulties are reconciled, we must ask what—if anything—does such a binary division do to help in the classification of speech disorders. If all that is wanted is a way of knowing what level of description is needed, then it is not very helpful, as a narrow transcription is needed to know the type of disorder. If, on the other hand, one actually wants to capture something about how the disorder operates within the patient's own speech component and so how to treat it, it has been shown that this division is insufficient.

We have pointed to problems with the classification into phonetic and phonological disorders from the output (i.e., speech) end. Several authors have noted also that a binary division cannot capture the input end of a speech problem. For example, Grunwell (1985) has pointed to the difference between a data-oriented and a speaker-oriented account of speech disorders, and Hewlett (1985) and Harris and Cottam (1985) both note that a two-way distinction is not sufficient to capture what may be happening at the input end of the speech process. For example, although phonological substitution patterns in a patient's speech may result from a disorder in the higher level organizational part of the subject's linguistic competence (in the "phonological component"), this is not always the case. Hewlett notes that a speaker may have the correct phonological contrast system in the phonological component and so "chose" the correct sound. However, the phonetic production system may be disordered so that what emerges is something that "sounds" like another phoneme (and may indeed be identical to it). This sort of disorder is, then, less a phonological one and more a particularly severe form of a phonetic disorder.

Hewlett gives an example with a target /s/. The first error type (termed "phonological" by that author) can be illustrated by the speaker choosing to produce the phoneme /t/ instead of /s/ and, indeed, uttering [t]. The second type ("phonetic") involves the choice of /s/, but a slight distortion of this results in the uttering of dental [s̪]. The third type ("articulatory") would see the choice of /s/ once more, but a greater distortion results in [t] being produced. Naturally, such a tripartite division is difficult to make purely from the transcription record. To tell whether a particular phonemic error is from phonological planning or a phonetic implementation problem, involves assessment of, for example, the patient's abilities in discrimination tests and the overall patterns of the patient's speech (see Hewlett, 1985, Hawkins, 1985).

The point about examining overall patterns in a patient's speech data is an important one. The small samples we have given above were chosen to illustrate individual points: naturally, in a real investigation much fuller information would be needed. We demonstrate the importance of this with the following transcriptions.

Speaker H. Target /s/.

so	[ʃoʊ]	soup	[ʃuːp]
sack	[ʃæk]	sea	[ʃiː]
sing	[ʃɪŋ]	some	[ʃʌm]

From these data it could be assumed that Speaker H is operating a phonological substitution of /s/ → [ʃ] and, therefore, that this does not involve any phonetic level distortions. However, the picture changes in looking at a transcription of a larger set of target words.

Speaker H. Target Alveolars.

so	[ʃoʊ]	soup	[ʃuːp]
sack	[ʃæk]	sea	[ʃiː]
sing	[ʃɪŋ]	some	[ʃʌm]
zoo	[ʒuː]	is	[ɪʒ]
two	[tʲuː]	ten	[tʲenʲ]
does	[dʲʌʒ]	need	[nʲiːdʲ]
net	[nʲetʲ]	noon	[nʲuːnʲ]

These data demonstrate that Speaker H actually has a pervasive process of palatalization that affects target alveolars. In the case of alveolar fricatives, this palatalization happens to result in palato-alveolar fricatives, with the plosives and nasals it results in palatalization as a secondary articulation. It is clear that we have a single phonetic level distortion with this speaker that looks like phonemic substitution with one group of sounds, but not when a larger set of data is included. This shows the need for care even in assigning the category of "phonological" error but, at least in such an instance, one can use phonetic transcription—of a *large* sample—to help decide on the correct analysis.

Some researchers have attempted to tie the idea of a three-way division of speech error types to different components within the language competence of speakers, and to relate impairments within these specific components to particular language pathologies. Code and Ball (1988) discuss this in some detail and here their conclusions are briefly summed up. Drawing on the work of several scholars, they identify three main components in the speech production process (though that does not necessarily mean there are only three such components). These are shown in the Figure 5–1. The diagram in Figure 5–1 has a phonological-type component at the top, with the utterance planned and the units of speech selected (including phonemes, assuming they exist at an abstract level, which is not accepted by all theorists). Below this is a cognitive phonetic component (described among others by Tatham [1984]), in which the planning for the implementation of the speech patterns is carried out. Finally, there is an articulatory phonetics component, with the actual motor activity taking place resulting in speech.

Although this is similar to the division proposed by Hewlett (1985), it is not identical. His division between phonetic and articulatory errors seems to be based more on the output rather than the input (i.e., more distortion may make an error seem phonological when it is not). With the Code and Ball (1988) analysis, we might claim that disturbances to the central conceptual component of language (as in aphasia) is likely to result in phonological error; disturbances at the phonetic planning stage may result in cognitive phonetic errors (as in apraxia of speech); and disturbances at the motor stage may result in articulatory phonetic errors (as in dysarthria). In fact, from the output point of view these last two types may appear, in some instances, to be very similar; the difference lies in the fact that motor errors are disorders in which the speaker is unable to produce a particular sound, with cognitive phonetic errors being those in which a patient is unable to plan a sound correctly in a particular context (but may well be able to produce it by imitation, etc.).

It has been shown, therefore, that phonetic transcription is only partially a help in determining error types. From a data-oriented viewpoint, one may be able to use transcription to identify errors that clearly involve phonological substitu-

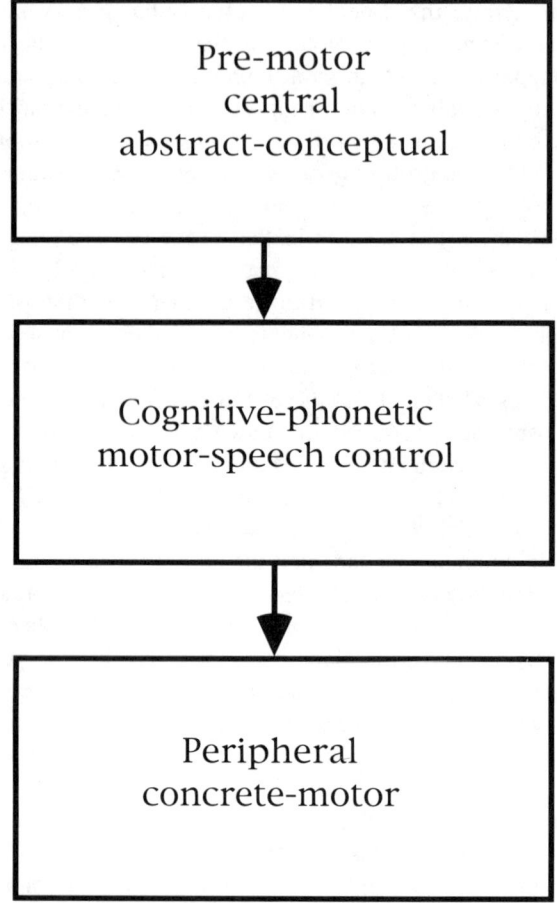

Figure 5–1. A three-way model of speech production.

tions if there is enough material on which to base one's analysis. However, if the errors do not appear to be purely phonological, one may need a knowledge of the patient's ability on other speech-related tasks before errors can be assigned to a purely phonetic category. Further, if one is interested in an input analysis, one will need to investigate which parts of the speech production process are impaired and which are intact before a judgment can be made.

Transcription as a Severity Measure

If transcription alone cannot be used as a way of classifying types of disorder, can it be used to measure how severe a disorder is? In a transcription consisting solely of phonological substitution patterns, a comparison between the number of phonological units (i.e., phonemes) in the target transcription and the number in the patient's realization may well work as a rough-and-ready measure of severity. This can be seen by examining the following examples. The first transcription set is that of the target pronunciation for the words listed; the second and third represent transcriptions of two different speakers with different degrees of severity in phonological disorders.

Set 1. Target Pronunciation

car	[kɑːɹ]	goat	[goʊt]
song	[sɒːŋ]	show	[ʃoʊ]
foot	[fʊt]	though	[ðoʊ]
goes	[goʊz]	vase	[veɪs]
think	[θɪŋk]	shake	[ʃeɪk]

The second transcription is of a speaker with a mild phonological disorder:

Speaker I.

car	[tɑːɹ]	goat	[doʊt]
song	[sɒːn]	show	[ʃoʊ]
foot	[fʊt]	though	[ðoʊ]
goes	[doʊz]	vase	[veɪs]
think	[θɪnt]	shake	[ʃeɪt]

This speaker has a total of 7 errors or errors on three different target phonemes.

Speaker J.

car	[tɑːɹ]	goat	[doʊt]
song	[tɒːn]	show	[toʊ]
foot	[pʊt]	though	[doʊ]
goes	[doʊd]	vase	[beɪt]
think	[tɪnt]	shake	[teɪt]

Speaker J, on the other hand, has a total of 16 errors or errors on 10 different target phonemes.

It would seem, then, that for phonological errors, a simple counting mechanism may well work as a measure of severity. However, one might ask what use such a measure is to the speech-language pathologist. The main analysis that is needed if adequate treatment is to be planned is one that illustrates what exactly is going wrong, not how many errors there are. In other words, measures such as 3 as opposed to 10 target phonemes being affected are less useful than those that tell us, for example, that velars are being fronted to alveolars in Speaker I, but that this process is added to in Speaker J by one that results in target fricatives being realized as plosives. Indeed, depending on the speech sample collected, the number of individual errors may be misleading and may not correlate with the number of phonological processes affecting the speaker.

If we turn to measuring severity in data that does not show phonological substitution patterns (or not these alone), it becomes more difficult to use transcription as a measure of severity. One can, of course, simply count the numbers of symbols that are not identical to the target sound as was done with the previous examples. However, this disguises that some distortions may well be thought of as more severe than others. For example, a subject who uses a dental articulation for an alveolar articulation throughout (i.e., /t, d, s, z, n, l/ → [t̪, d̪, s̪, z̪, n̪, l̪]) is not going to cause any perceptual confusion and such a distortion must be considered minor. On the other hand, a speaker using [ɬ, ɭ] for /s, z/ may still maintain a contrast with other fricatives, but the sounds are going to be perceived as markedly unnatural, and so we would want to score them as somehow a more severe disorder than the dentalization process.

One possible solution might be to count diacritic use separately from symbol use. That is to say, considering the addition of a diacritic as being less severe a disorder than the use of a totally different symbol. This can work in practice as:

Speaker K.

see	[s̪iː]	she	[çiː]
so	[s̪oʊ]	show	[çoʊ]
said	[s̪ed]	shed	[çed]

These data demonstrate a minor change of articulation (from alveolar to dental, but still maintaining the same part of the tongue in the articulation) in the case of target /s/, but a more severe problem with target /ʃ/, as in this instance not only is there a change in place of articulation, but the part of the tongue involved in producing the fricative is also different. This difference is reflected in the choice of diacritic rather than symbol. However, not all examples fit neatly into this distinction:

Speaker L.

tie	[taɪ]	fly	[ɸlaɪ]
do	[duː]	if	[ɪɸ]
night ·	[naɪt̼]	veep	[βiːp]
lid	[l̼ɪd]	love	[lʌβ]

This sample also has some sounds with diacritics added to the target symbols and some shown with different symbols. However, in this case, one would surely want to argue that a linguo-labial articulation (e.g., [t̼]) is considerably less usual (and so more severe a disorder) than the slight difference between bilabial and labiodental articulations.

It is becoming clear, therefore, that some of the differences in transcription between the use of diacritics and symbols is an artifact of the symbol system being used; in other words, the existence of symbols or diacritics for a particular articulation is often (though not always) an accident of history rather than a reflection of real phonetic differences. A further example makes this clear:

Speaker M.

pet	[pet]	man	[ŋæn]
but	[b̪ʌt]	may	[ɱeɪ]
cup	[kʌp̪]	some	[sʌɱ]
tub	[tʌb̪]	game	[geɪɱ]

If we were to assume that diacritics scored more severely than symbols then, for *these* data, we would be forced to say that the distortions of target /m/ are worse than those for target /p, b/. However, both sets are obviously showing a process of converting bilabials into labiodentals; it just so happens that there is a specific symbol in the IPA for a labiodental nasal, but to show labiodental plosives we have to make use of a diacritic (as recommended in the extIPA symbols).

Examples of the Transcription
of Disordered Speech

In this final chapter part we illustrate some uses of phonetic transcription with a variety of speech disorders. We provide some typical transcriptions using both IPA and extIPA symbols, only covering some of the features likely to be encountered in a selection of speech disorder types. We do not include any prosodic

information or disorders where suprasegmental features are the most salient errors encountered, as these are dealt with in Chapter 7. Further, we are most interested here in illustrating what we have termed "phonetic" disorders, rather than those where phonological substitutions are the norm. In the five cases presented, we concentrate on child speech, although we do include one example of an adult dysarthric speaker.

Misarticulations in Child Speech

There are, of course, a wide variety of misarticulations encountered in child speech; here we illustrate three cases.

Case 1

This child has a general fronting process that results in some phonemic substitution patterns, but others where atypical sounds are utilized.

thin	[θ̞ɪn]	so	[s̪oʊ]
cat	[tæt̪]	foot	[ɸʊt̪]
shop	[sɒːp]	dog	[d̪ɒːd]
both	[boʊθ̞]	tease	[t̪iːz̟]
that	[ð̥æt̪]	goose	[duːs]

The fronting does not result, however, in the loss of phonemic contrastivity, although the speech sounds very disturbed. Therapeutic intervention in this case should take into account the desirability of maintaining these phonological contrasts; therefore, the establishment of a velar place of articulation should take precedence over moving the linguolabial articulations back to alveolar.

Case 2

This child exhibits what is commonly termed a lisp. However, the detailed transcription shows that two distinct lisp types are exhibited, which again maintain phonological contrastivity.

sip	[ɬɪp]	zip	[ɮɪp]
hiss	[hɪɬ]	his	[hɪɮ]
racer	[ɹeɪɬɚ]	razor	[ɹeɪɮɚ]
stop	[ɬtɑːp]	lost	[lɒːɬt]
spy	[ɬpaɪ]	buzzed	[bʌɮd]

ship	[ʂɪp]	hush	[hʌɬ]
pressure	[pɹeɬɚ]	pleasure	[pleɮɚ]
wished	[wɪɬt]	garage	[gəɹɑːɮ]

Although target alveolar fricatives are realized as alveolar lateral fricatives, target palato-alveolars are realized as combined median and lateral fricatives. Auditorily, these may sound very similar, but it is clear the child does maintain a phonological contrast. Therefore, therapy should concentrate on achieving correct articulator placement rather than working at a phoneme level.

Case 3

This case concerns the overuse of a lip-shape harmonization process. Here, alveolar contexts produce a lip-spreading process, while labial, palato-alveolar and velar contexts produce a lip-rounding process. These processes affect both consonants and vowels.

ten	[ten]	two	[tɯː]
nod	[nɑːd]	loose	[lɯːs]
peep	[pyːp]	keep	[kʷyːp]
beam	[byːm]	gang	[gʷœŋʷ]
sheep	[ʃʷyːp]	rip	[ɹʷʏp]

When both alveolar and non-alveolar sounds are present in the word, progressive assimilation is seen.

tube	[tyːb]	dog	[dɑːg]
sheet	[ʃʷyːtʷ]	read	[ɹʷyːdʷ]
green	[gʷɹʷyːnʷ]	bead	[byːdʷ]

Clearly, this case is quite complex, and therapy will have to concentrate on divorcing the lip-posture from the place of articulation.

Cleft Palate or Velopharyngeal Inadequacy

The data for this case are adapted from Howard (1993, pp. 307–309).

Case 4

| baby | [b̃eɪbɪ] | toy | [ʔɔɪ] |
| cat | [ʔæʔʰ] | tap | [ʔæʔⵔ] |

paper	[p͡ʔeɪp̰ʔə]	kick	[ʔɪʔʰ]
bucket	[b̰ʊʔɪʔʰ]	Sue	[ç̰u]
Daddy	[ʔæʔɪ]	dog	[ʔɒʔʰ]
sugar	[ɕ̰ɭʊʔə]	shoe	[ç̰ʷu]

These data illustrate the child's realization of place contrasts. It is interesting that, although these pronunciations are often markedly deviant from the target, they manage in many cases to maintain contrastivity. So, although alveolars are most often realized by glottal stops for plosives, bilabials retain some kind of bilabial aspects. Velars, however, are not regularly distinguished from alveolars. The following data also show that alveolar and palato-alveolar targets are usually contrasted, as are plosives, fricatives, and affricates, as well as approximants, at least in word-initial position.

tap	[ʔæʔↃ]	down	[ʔaʊɴ]
chair	[ʔjeə]	jam	[ʔjæm]
sock	[ç̰ɒʔʰ]	shop	[ç̰ʷjɒp̰ʰ]
zip	[ç̰ɪʔↃ]	cup	[ʔʊʔʰ]
go	[ʔəʊ]	yes	[jɛʔ]
why	[waɪ]	letter	[ɥḛʔə]
glasses	[ɴwæ̰ç̰ə̰ç̰]	ring	[ʊɪɴ]

The nasal-oral contrast was usually maintained, although again not often according to the target norms. In fact, the following data demonstrate that a uvular nasal is used for both alveolar and velar nasal targets (bilabial nasals having been satisfactorily established during therapy) in contrast to the glottal stop or bilabial plosives (again these latter having been worked on in therapy) used for the oral stops.

letter	[ɥḛʔə]	nose	[ɴəʊç̰]
ladder	[ɥæʔə]	ring	[ʊɪɴ]
sugar	[ɕ̰ɭʊʔə]	fine	[f̰ːaɪɴ]
down	[ʔaʊɴ]	penny	[p̰ʔeɴɪ]
dog	[ʔɒʔʰ]	singing	[ç̰ɪɴɪɴ]
cat	[ʔæʔʰ]	teaspoon	[ʔɪ̰ç̰b̰uɴ]
pig	[Ↄɪʔʰ]	mud	[məʔʰ]
pen	[ʔeɴ]	mum	[məm]
tap	[ʔæʔↃ]	mouth	[maʊθ]
paper	[p͡ʔeɪp̰ʔə]	thumb	[θəm]

big	[mɪʔʰ]	jam	[ʔjæm]
baby	[b̃eɪbɪ]	hammer	[h̃æmə]

These data also demonstrate the child's general success with the dental fricatives.

Finally, one can consider this child's ability with the voicing contrast. As the above data have shown, this contrast is very often not apparent, surfacing only with labials: the bilabial plosives and sometimes with the labio-dental fricatives. Below we show some examples in which the voicing contrast is maintained.

pig	[ɵɪʔʰ]	bib	[b̃ɪb̥ʰ]
four	[fɔ]	a van	[ə f̬æɴ]
feather	[f̩eʋə]	laughing	[æf̩ɪɴ]

The speaker uses a click or simultaneous voiceless bilabial plus glottal stop to mark initial /p/, employing some kind of voiced bilabial stops (usually plus nasal escape) to mark /b/. With the labiodental fricatives, the voiceless fricative is realized as a weakly articulated fricative, with the voiced target produced as a strongly articulated fricative or an approximant.

This case shows markedly deviant pronunciations, but also the importance of accurate and detailed transcriptions—not only to demonstrate the articulatory strategies adopted by this particular subject, but also to highlight those areas where contrastivity is maintained and those where it is lost.

Dysarthria

The data for this case are adapted from Ball, Code, Rahilly, and Hazlett (1994). In the transcript, "T" stands for the therapist, and "W" for the patient.

Case 5

T: just ask you to say a few phrases . . . open the door

W: [{$_{lento}$ V̰!! oʊ ʔən ə d̥ɛ: V̰!! $_{lento}$ }]

T: close the window

W: [{$_{lento}$ V̰!! hloʊh ə wɪnd̥oʊ V!! $_{lento}$ }]

T: wash the dishes

W: [{$_{lento}$ V̰!! wɒh ə ʔɪhɪhɪ: V̰!! $_{lento}$ }]

The transcription for subject W uses several prosodic symbols for marking voice quality that are fully explained in later chapters; nevertheless, the use of weakly articulated segments, deletion of certain initial sounds, and a weakening of fricatives to [h] can be noted. As is often the case with dysarthria, there is what can be termed a pervasive lenition in operation, and therapy will have to concentrate on strengthening of articulation as well as attempting to alter the voice quality settings used by the subject.

Conclusion

In this chapter we have illustrated the importance of transcription to the proper understanding (and therefore treatment) of disordered speech with a wide range of examples. Of course, sometimes patients' speech is so nonnormal that even competent phoneticians find it difficult to transcribe. This, however, does not mean that such cases should be left untranscribed. Indeed, the more disrupted the speech, the more important it is to find out about it. In such cases, though, one may need to access other information, such as that available from instrumental analysis, to aid the description. We return to this point in more detail in Chapter 9.

CHAPTER

6

The Transcription of Prosody

Prosodic Features and Syllables

Prosody covers features of pronunciation that are of a quite different order from consonants and vowels. Imagine a person in danger from drowning in a river who cries out "Help!" and another who is hosting a buffet lunch who quietly encourages a guest "Help yourself; please don't wait to be asked." The two people have both used the word *help* and in both situations that word would be transcribed /help/. However, there is a tremendous difference in the actual articulation of that word in the two circumstances. What are the differences?

Firstly, the cry for help will be much louder than the polite offer at the buffet lunch. The volume of air expelled from the lungs will be vastly greater, the cry will involve a much greater degree of muscular effort, and the vocal folds will be opened to a much greater extent during the vibration process.

Secondly, the cry for help will begin at a much higher pitch of voice. The cry will probably be characterized by a high pitch for as long as possible before it begins to trail off to a lower pitch. As the expelled air passes through the larynx, the vocal folds will vibrate at a much faster rate than they would for the polite offer.

Thirdly, the cry for help will last a lot longer than the polite offer. The host who says "Help yourself" will say the word *help* quite quickly; whereas the person in danger of drowning is likely to extend the articulation of the word for several seconds.

So, although the broad transcription of *help* would be identical in the two cases, one is well aware of other features that accompany the four segments. These differences in loudness, pitch and length are generally known as the prosodic features. The origin of the term *prosody* is the Greek verb "to sing with"; thus, these three features are thought of as "accompanying" the consonants and vowels. An alternative term that has been used is *suprasegmental*, in that these features are above the segments, they belong to a unit of structure that is larger than the segment. The prosodic, or suprasegmental, features are characteristic of *syllables*. So it would be more accurate to talk about loud or high-pitched syllables, rather than loud or high-pitched consonants and vowels. As it happens, length is often attributed to consonants and vowels: the vowel in the English word *bead* is inherently longer than that in the word *bid*, but its length correlates directly with the articulatory feature of tongue muscular tension. Length of articulation can also characterize the production of consonants; for instance, the final /m/ of *Mom* is noticeably longer than the initial /m/. However, in addition to length of time in the articulation of consonants and vowels, length is also a characteristic feature of syllables—as in the above example of /help/—and is thus also considered a prosodic feature.

These two functions of length, as in articulations of segments and in syllables, illustrate the two functions fulfilled by the three prosodic features. Loudness, pitch and length are used both linguistically and paralinguistically. The example of the two instances in which *help* is used illustrates the paralinguistic function of prosody. Paralanguage is the social, or cultural, system that indicates something about the messenger rather than the message; in speech, it corresponds to what is commonly called the "tone of voice," which expresses something of how a speaker is feeling while giving a message. The linguistic use of prosody, on the other hand, relates to the message itself; typically, it differentiates between words, such as length being one distinctive feature between /iː/ and /ɪ/, thus "making a bead" is a different message from "making a bid"; and *wholly* is a different lexical item from *holy* because of its longer /l/; and differences in prosody are responsible for differences in phrases and whole utterances. Consider, for instance, the ambiguity of the utterance *it's hot, isn't it* with either a falling or a rising pitch of the voice on the tag *isn't it*.

Prosody is important. Thus whenever speech is being recorded, or transcribed, onto paper, prosodic features must be indicated.

There are five principles to be noted in any discussion of the transcription of prosody:

1. Prosodic features are relative, not absolute. This is most clearly illustrated in the case of pitch. The exact pitch of *help* in the case of the person in danger of drowning and of the host at the buffet lunch depends on who the person is; generally speaking, voice pitch of women is higher than that of men, and the voice pitch of children is higher than that of women. Thus, it is not difficult to imagine a child's low pitch being higher, in absolute musical terms, than a man's high pitch. When we transcribe aspects of pitch, or length, or loudness, then we do so in relative terms to the general profile of the speaker. One person's long vowel might well be shorter than another person's short vowel, simply because the second person's natural speaking rate is slower.

2. Prosodic features are features of syllables. It is the syllable as a whole that is stressed or high pitched, not its constituent phonemes. Length is a feature of both segments and syllables.

3. Prosodic features are present in every utterance, and therefore, in every language. The utterance *hold your horses* happens to contain no nasal articulation, for example, but every utterance must contain some degree of loudness, even if it is very soft; likewise, no utterance can be made without pitch (unless it is whispered); even a monotone is spoken on a particular pitch; and every utterance occupies a timespan, however rapidly spoken. Even if the utterance consists of a solitary syllable with a single vowel, such as a hesitational /ə/, it must be accompanied by some degree of loudness, pitch and length.

4. Prosodic features are systematic. Because they are ever present, all languages engage them, but different languages exploit them in different ways. An obvious example is the case of pitch in so-called tone languages. Many languages of the world employ differences of pitch to distinguish lexical items; a good example is the Thai language. If the word /khaː/ is spoken on a mid pitch, it means (Tingsabadh & Abramson, 1993, p. 26) "to get stuck," but with a falling pitch, it means "I"; with a high pitch, it means "trade"; with a low pitch, it means "kill," and with a rising pitch, "leg." There is nothing that corresponds to this use of pitch in English; for instance, if you pronounced the English word *no* in the five different ways specified for in Thai, it will mean "no" every time: the contribution that each of the five ways of saying *no* makes to a conversation will be different, but the basic meaning of the word does not change, as it would using the Thai example. English makes use of a combination of all three features to make some syllables more prominent, or salient, than others; a syllable that combines a greater degree of loudness, a higher degree of pitch, and greater length will stand out from relatively quieter, lower pitched, and shorter syllables. Compare the prominence of the two identically segmented syllables of the English word *cocoa* /kəʊkəʊ/; the first is more prominent than the second and this is captured by saying that the first syllable is stressed while the second is unstressed.

5. Prosodic features operate as the basic constituents of word stress, tone (in tone languages), rhythm, and intonation. Rhythm covers the characteristic combinations of more and less prominent syllables and is thus the product of prosodic features. Intonation is primarily the sequence of variously pitched syllables forming a tune or melody, and is thus also the product of prosodic features. The combination of all three features as the constituents of English word stress, and the special use of pitch for lexical tone in tone languages have been mentioned. Thus, in many languages, a prosodic feature or a combination of features functions at the level of word phonology, by identifying one word as distinct from another. Take another example from English, the sequence of segments /ɪnsaɪt/; which word is it, *insight* or *incite*? Without some indication of the prosodic features, it is impossible to tell.

It must now be conceded that a transcription devoid of the notation of prosodic features is inadequate; at best, it is ambiguous.

The importance of syllables is related to their function of being the relevant units for carrying the prosodic features, and thus being the basic unit of word stress systems, tone in tone languages, rhythm, and intonation. There is another aspect of their importance: the terms *consonant* and *vowel* are defined in terms of their respective functions within the syllable, and the distribution of consonant and vowel phonemes and their allophonic varieties are dictated according to positions in the syllable.

The occurrence of certain allophonic manifestations at a particular point in a syllable is sometimes crucial in distinguishing between two words. A well-known example employs the words *nitrate* and *night-rate*. Superficially, they have an identical sequence of segments: /naɪtreɪt/. However, native speakers pronounce them quite distinctly, by dividing the sequence differently into two syllables: the first would be /naɪ/ and /treɪt/, the second /naɪt/ and /reɪt/. It is the syllable division that is crucial for interpretation. The middle /t/ of *nitrate* is aspirated to such an extent that it devoices the following /r/; the middle /t/ of *night-rate* is quite likely to be unreleased and, therefore, not aspirated or to be replaced entirely by a glottal stop; in either case, the /r/ is left fully voiced. Furthermore, the (diphthongal) vowel in the first syllable of *nitrate* is fully long, as it would be in an open syllable, but the equivalent vowel in *night-rate* is shortened (or "clipped") as a consequence of a following fortis, voiceless, consonant. This combination of allophonic features constitutes differences of juncture between the segments in sequence, and because the identity of the location of the syllable division is crucial, it needs to be recorded in transcription.

However, it is not often in English that juncture at syllable boundaries is crucial, but where it is—to distinguish between two possible interpretations—it needs to be noted. Gimson (1989, pp. 304–306) described the junctural details of the following potentially ambiguous examples:

piːstɔːks	(pea stalks/peace talks)
ə neɪm	(a name/an aim)
ðætstʌf	(that stuff/that's tough)

ðə weɪtəkʌtɪt	(the way to cut it/the waiter cut it)[1]
aɪskriːm	(I scream/ice cream)
haʊstreɪnd	(how strained/housetrained)
waɪtʃuːz	(why choose/white shoes)

A variety of conventions have been used in which it has been felt necessary to indicate the boundary between two syllables. Jones (1957), Westermann and Ward (1933) and Cruttenden (1986, p. xiv) used the hyphen for this purpose, for example:

toe strap	'tou-stræp
mouse trap	'maus-træp

(Jones, 1957, p. 327)

ŋgom	one syllable
ŋ-gom	two syllables
ŋ-go-m	three syllables

(Westermann & Ward, 1933, p. 111)

Trager (1964) used the double cross [#] to indicate different junctures between syllables, equivalent to the use of the hyphen. Bailey (1985) preferred the use of the tilde [~], as in ['lɔ˞-yə] for *lawyer* (p. 17). J. Wells (1990) simply uses a letter space (see the *Stress* section below for examples).

However, the most widely used symbol for syllable division is the dot, or period [.], see Abercrombie (1967), Ladefoged (1982), K. L. Pike (1947) and the IPA:

lightning	'laɪt.nɪŋ
lightening	'laɪt.n̩.ɪŋ (Ladefoged, 1982, p. 223)

It should also be noted that dictionaries use a similar range of devices to indicate the boundaries of syllables: hyphens (Hawkins, 1982) and raised dots

---

[1]This example only works with non-rhotic accents, those in which the final "'r" of "waiter" would not be pronounced.

(Hornby, 1989). However, it should also be noted that the boundaries indicated usually relate to spelling, and not to pronunciation.

Pausing

Pausing is the absence of articulation. It is not necessarily equivalent to silence. The difference in meaning of two renderings of the phrase *old men and women*, is effected by a change of rhythm: if there is a pause after *men*, the "domain" of *old* is restricted to *men*, with the implication that the *women* referred to are not old. The pause itself may be absolutely silent or it may be "filled" by a lengthening of the vowel and final consonant of *men*.

1. oldmenandwomen (no break = both men and women referred to are old)
2. (a) oldmen І І andwomen (silent pause after *men* = only men referred to are old)
    (b) oldme-n-andwomen (filled pause after *men* = only men referred to are old)

It should also be noted that the pause in this case fits in rhythmically with the articulation of the whole phrase; hesitations, on the other hand, usually interrupt and distort the rhythm of articulation.

The pause that distinguishes the two possible meanings of *old men and women* performs a grammatical function: It restricts the domain of the adjective to the first noun. There are many examples in the grammar of English of this function of pause; either at the level of phrases:

put it on the table in the middle	(either "the table which is in the middle" or "in the middle of the table")
fight with the ambulancemen	(either "against them" or "alongside them")
they climbed on to the top	(either "onto" = preposition or "on" = element of phrasal verb *to climb on*, "carry on climbing")

or as the marker of intonation unit boundaries:

my brother who lives in Derby	(either, identifying which brother or adding supplementary information on the one brother)
they didn't come because of the money	(either, "they came, but not because of the money" or "they didn't come" with a reason given)

Pausing has other functions besides grammatical. Pausing can help to support emphasis, as in:

the most I I awful thing has happened

It also helps to indicate the end of somebody's turn in conversation or monologue:

and that ends children's programs I I for today
well I I that's all I I I I want to talk about I I this morning

Pausing can also be a rhetorical device, as in changes of pace, intended to keep the listeners' interest or to impress them with a particular point:

well I I that's not I I quite I I what I had I I in mind

The grammatical, emphatic, terminal, and rhetorical functions of pausing all involve an extra rhythmical beat, whether the pauses are literally silent or "filled."

Hesitations, on the other hand, do usually interrupt the rhythm of speech. They are occasioned by searching for a word, by correcting a mispronunciation, or by abandoning a grammatical structure in favour of another. Here is an example from Crystal and Davy (1975, p. 19):

he's I I he's been to the la I I to oh I I the last f f two or three world cup I I world cup I I mat things you know I I tournaments I I

What is striking about these cases of hesitation pauses is that they do not occur at predictable points of syntax and that they clearly disturb the rhythm.

Hesitations are a normal, inevitable characteristic of unrehearsed, spontaneous speech. As Brown, Currie and Kenworthy pointed out, hesitations are hardly surprising:

> In producing spontaneous speech the speaker has to decide on a topic, select the "staging" procedures for presenting his topic . . . determine what he must introduce as new and what he can take as given, sort out the appropriate syntactic structures, select lexical items, check that his listener is following what he is saying and agreeing with it, make it clear that he wishes to continue with or to give away his turn, quite apart from speaking. (Brown, Currie, & Kenworthy, 1980, p. 47)

Whether pausing fulfils grammatical, emphatic, terminal, or rhetorical functions or is the product of hesitation, it is important to be aware that it occurs very frequently in speech and needs to be recorded in transcription.

Pausing has been marked in several ways. Halliday (1970) and Abercrombie (1971) used the caret [∧] to indicate a silent beat, to illustrate, for example, the difference between old men and women

and

old men ʌ and women

K. L. Pike (1945, 1947) distinguished between tentative and final pauses in relation to intonation and used either single or double slashes [/], [//] (1945) or single or double bars [|], [| |] (1947). Both pause types vary in length; "the tentative pause is usually shorter in length than the final one, but it is not always so." (K. L. Pike 1945, p. 31). Thus K. L. Pike distinguishes between two functions of pause within an utterance, rather than between degrees of pause length.

Crystal (1969) distinguished between four degrees of silent pause: a unit pause ("the interval of an individual's rhythm cycle from one prominent syllable (arsis) to the next, within a stable tempo," Crystal 1969, p. 171), double and treble pause, and a brief pause ("a silence perceivably shorter than (and usually approximately half as long) as unit length," p. 171). He also drew attention to two types of voiced pause: brief and unit. In Crystal and Davy (1969), four lengths of voiced pause were also mentioned. Their symbols are:

Pause	silent	voiced
unit	-	əː(m)
double	--	əːəː
treble	----	əːəːəː
brief	.	ə(m)

Later, in Crystal and Davy (1975), in the publication of transcribed conversational extracts, they retained the notation for silent pauses, but spelled the voiced pauses as *er, erm, m*.

Brown et al. (1980) made use of the plus sign [+] for a brief pause, and double plus [++] for longer pauses but added the actual timing of such pauses:

> I regret + putting the people out of the out of the South Side and Central Edinburgh you know ++ 0.86 I don't think ++ 1.8 especially after the war you know. (Brown et al., 1980, p. 66)

The timing of pauses became accepted practice in the transcription of conversation and provided scholars like Lehiste (1982) with evidence for the marking of phonological paragraphs and conversational turns (see Chapter 7).

There are no recognized IPA symbols for pausing. Duckworth et al. (1990) reporting the extIPA symbols recommended dots, or periods, within parentheses:[2]

---

[2]The periods are placed within parentheses to avoid confusion with IPA diacritics.

x(.)x	short pause
x(..)x	medium-length pause
x(...)x	long pause

Otherwise, Crystal and Davy's system is recommended.

Voice Quality

The production of voice, phonation, has, like the prosodic features, both linguistic and paralinguistic dimensions to its use. The linguistic dimension inevitably affects the phonological system itself, with the paralinguistic dimension expressing characteristics of the speaker. The linguistic dimension includes the distinction between voiced and voiceless articulations. Inherently different symbol shapes represent this voice distinction between consonants; the distinction between voiced and voiceless vowels is indicated by a diacritic or [h].

Vowels, in their normal, or unmarked, form are voiced; hence, a single diacritic can indicate a marked form like voicelessness. There are other marked forms; these other phonation types include whisper, creak, and breathiness. It is commonly agreed (Abercrombie, 1967, pp. 89–95; Catford, 1988, pp. 51–56; Clark &Yallop, 1990, pp. 59–61) that there are five typical phonation types: voice, voicelessness, whisper, creak and breathy voice. Each of these can enter into the phonological system of a language and either be distinctive features between phoneme systems or allophonic variations in the distribution of phonemes. On either count, there is a need to include them in a written record of speech.

Breathy voice, for instance, distinguishes one set of vowels from another in Dinka, a language of Sudan, and is the basis of the so-called aspirated voiced stops of many languages of India. Similarly, creaky voice distinguishes one set of vowels from another in several indigenous languages of Mexico. Whisper is, technically, the feature that distinguishes voiceless vowels from voiced in many languages.

However, there is also a broader use of voice qualities. Instead of a single segment or a defined sequence of segments being distinguished by a particular phonation type, whole utterances can be affected. This is obviously the case in whispered speech: Creaky voice can permeate whole utterances if the speaker is tired, or ill, breathy voice is the product of great physical exertion affecting speech, such as speaking after or while running.

Apart from such purely physical constraints on speech, there is a more strictly social dimension in paralanguage. Creaky voice often accompanies low-pitched articulation, particularly at final intonation boundaries and may give an impression of seriousness and authority. Breathy quality may be employed to produce a husky voice, with sexual overtones.

There is also another type of muscular control over phonation that also affects speech at large, namely register. Register refers to types of phonation in respect to pitch. A person's normal speech and normal range of pitch control operate in what is generally known as chest register. Falsetto register operates at a much higher range of pitch, above the highest pitch normally attainable by chest register. Singing requires a different register again, known as middle voice register (discussed in Clark & Yallop, 1990, p. 41).

The term "voice quality" was also used by Abercrombie (1967, pp. 91–95) for a wider range of speech effects than just phonation types; he used it to refer to, "those characteristics that are present more or less all the time that a person is talking; it is a quasi-permanent quality running through all the sound that issues from his mouth" (Abercrombie, 1967, p. 91).

Certain characteristics are "fixed," being outside a speaker's control. Some characteristics are temporary, due to medical conditions like tonsillitis, laryngitis, the common cold, enlarged adenoids, and so on. Other characteristics are permanent and derive from the fine variations of the anatomy of the individual; these characteristics can be termed "indexical" because they identify an individual's voice. Strikingly obvious variations identify the age and the sex of a speaker. Because these components lie outside a person's control, they cannot be used to convey meaning, linguistically.

Other characteristics lie within a person's control, although some may be acquired unconsciously. An example of conscious control over a speech characteristic is the pursing of the lips, which is typical of speech directed to a baby; this gives a continuous overall labialization effect to such utterances. Utterances could be characterized similarly with constant palatalization or constant velarization, or by any such secondary articulation. It is also quite conceivable that a person may unconsciously adapt to a prevalent dialect feature like permanent nasal quality. The speakers of a particular language or dialect may be characterized by a particular articulatory setting acquired unconsciously by native speakers, but may be consciously acquired by a learner.

Voice qualities that are directly incorporated into a phonological system with either phonemic, or allophonic, status will clearly need to be identified in a written record of speech. Features such as chest register and those that lie outside speakers' control need not be identified other than as a general label, such as, *male, aged 40, laryngitis*. Then, depending on the purpose of a particular transcription, other qualities may or may not need recording for whole or part utterances.

The main tradition in transcribing voicelessness has been the use of a small subscript circle [̥], as in the following:

i̥ = voiceless front close unrounded vowel

r̥ = voiceless alveolar trill

However, Boas (1916), K. L. Pike (1945), and Smalley (1963) established an early American alternative by using capital letter equivalents of letters representing "normally" voiced sounds; thus the above two sounds were transcribed as [I] and [R], respectively. However, this practice inevitably but unnecessarily increased the number of phonetic symbols; it would also lead to confusion with similar symbols used in the IPA alphabet. Although Boas's practice had the merit of being typable, the resultant transcription looked ungainly.

Another advantage of the [̥] is its potential for indicating devoicing by being placed slightly to the left to indicate the delay in the onset of voicing during an articulation, and to the right the premature cessation of voicing (Wells, personal communication); thus,

$$\text{{}_{\circ}}b = \text{delayed onset in voicing}$$

$$b_{\circ} = \text{premature cessation}$$

Breathy voicing has been symbolized by various means including a superscript apostrophe and a subscript plus sign, [i'] and [i̟], but the current standard symbol established by IPA is a subscript pair of dots:

$$\underset{..}{i} = \text{breathy front close unrounded vowel}$$

$$\underset{..}{r} = \text{breathy voiced alveolar trill}$$

Creaky voicing has also been symbolized by various means including a superscript glottal stop symbol, [i $^{?}$], but the current standard symbol established by IPA is a subscript tilde:

$$\underset{\sim}{i} = \text{creaky (laryngealized) front close unrounded vowel}$$

$$\underset{\sim}{r} = \text{creaky voiced alveolar trill}$$

Before leaving the general theme of voice quality, it would be as well to acknowledge other types of activity that impinge on speech. Although we are talking, we often engage in activities that are directly related to the message we are sharing and that directly effect our speech, such as laughter, giggle, sighing, sobbing—reactions that involve tremulousness in the voice, and so on. These involuntary physical reflexes of emotional states are not, strictly, part of paralanguage, but because they will have a noticeable effect on speech, it may be necessary to make reference to the given speech effect.

Stress

Prosodic features lend themselves to iconic notation systems to a greater extent than segmental features which in literate societies are inevitably tied to conventional orthographies. Prosody, though linguistically significant, has not been institutionalized orthographically in every culture; for instance, stress contrasts in English are not part of the language's spelling, as in Spanish. An acute accent marks the placement of stress in the Spanish *término* ("end") and *terminó* ("he or she finished") in contrast to its more typical placement in the penultimate syllable, *termino* ("I finish").

An iconic system represents a phonetic feature in a visual way. A stressed syllable, being more prominent than an unstressed syllable, can be represented in a relatively more prominent visual fashion, either by the size, shape, or heaviness of type or by some identifying mark. Length can similarly be represented iconically, such as by a longer or doubled symbol; and pitch can be represented by marks that spread themselves up and down a scale.

Sweet (1877) identified a stressed syllable by a raised dot following the vowel syllable: [a•]; this was known as a "turned period." Extra stress was identified by doubling the dot: [a••]. A half stress, or secondary stress, was indicated by the addition of a lower dot: [a:].

The Oxford English Dictionary (1933) followed a similar practice. The doubled "turned period" was used to indicate the primary accent of a compound, such as *a••fter-cou•nsel*. The dictionary employed the breve (˘) to indicate an "obscure" vowel, a vowel in an unstressed syllable that was reduced to /ə/. The following words were transcribed in the 1933 OED as follows :

Academic	(ækăde•mik)
Academical	(ækăde•mikăl)
Academically	(ækăde•mikăli)
Academician	(ăkæ:demi•ʃăn)
Academy	(ăkæ•dĕmi)

However, a different system emerged in the *Concise Oxford Dictionary of Current English* (1951). Stress was indicated by an acute accent /´/ after the syllable concerned. In this way, its inherent prominence was highlighted but at a point that indicated the prominence of the whole syllable, not just the vowel. The breve, though, was not used for an unstressed "obscure" vowel, but for a short vowel in either a stressed or unstressed syllable. The unstressed neutral vowel was not indicated at all, although a superscript dot over *e* indicated unstressed /ɪ/ such as *collė++ge*, *privė++t*. The very different function of the breve led to much confusion, but the system was intended to avoid phonetic respelling as far as possible, yielding:

> ăcadĕm´ic
>
> ăcadĕm´ical
>
> ăcadĕm´ĭ cally
>
> acăd´emi´cian (-shn)
>
> Acăd´emў

Oxford later produced a new generation of dictionaries for schools, exemplified by *The Oxford Senior Dictionary* (1982), in which a more directly iconic system for marking the pronunciation of stress was used. Stress was highlighted by bold type for the whole syllable. The breve indicated the unstressed neutral value. The pronunciation of many words was felt to be self-evident and was thus not indicated at all:

> academic   (ak-ă-**dem**-ik)
>
> academician   (ă-kad-ĕ-**mish**-ăn)
>
> academy

Finally, Oxford produced dictionaries for learners of English with a very different policy for supplying pronunciation information. The most famous has been the *Oxford Advanced Learners' Dictionary of Current English* (1989), in which the symbols of the IPA have always been used. Stress has always been indicated by the conventional IPA superior vertical stroke ['] before the syllable concerned, and an inferior equivalent for a secondary stress. The following transcriptions are the product of this policy:

> academic   /ˌækəˈdemɪk/
>
> academically   /-klɪ/
>
> academician   /əˌkædəˈmɪʃən; US ˌækədəˈmɪʃn/
>
> academy   /əˈkædəmɪ/
>
> Aˌcademy Aˈward

This policy has now also been adopted in the revised edition of the Oxford English Dictionary and appears to have gained acceptance by many other British dictionary publishers.

Webster's Third New International Dictionary of the English Language (1961) had already adopted the same convention

ac•a•demic	\'akə¦demik\
ac•a•de•mi•cian	\akə'də͵mishən\
ac•a•dem•i•cism	\akə'demə͵sizəm\
acad•e•mist	\ə'kadəməst\
acad•e•my	\ə'kadəmē\

The simultaneous primary and secondary stress marks in *academic* above indicate variation between the two degrees of stress.

It is, of course, possible to discriminate more degrees of stress than primary, secondary, and no stress. As Gimson (1989, p. 224) pointed out, in a word such as *examination,* it might be possible to detect a distinction in the degree of articulatory energy in each of the five syllables: "the syllables may be articulated with the following descending order of energy /neɪ/, /zæ/, /ɪg/, /mɪ/, /ʃn/" (p. 224). Nevertheless, native speakers generally only distinguish between stressed and unstressed syllables.

However, Gimson (1989, pp. 225, 229) did distinguish between two types of secondary stress: One is rhythmic as it carries a rhythmic beat distinct from that of the primary stress, but normally carries no pitch movement (as the primary stress does); the other is non-rhythmic and usually occurs immediately after the primary stress. The former is exemplified in the word *examination* /ɪg͵zæmɪ'neɪʃn/ where the second syllable, /͵zæ/, carries a beat; the latter is exemplified in the word *tobacco* /tə'bæ͵kəʊ/, where /͵kəʊ/ carries no beat.

Gimson distinguishes the two types of secondary stress by different symbols in an iconic representation of word stress patterns: the rhythmic second stress by a large solid dot and the nonrhythmic by a "hollow" dot of the same size. Primary stress was indicated by a large solid dot surmounted with a downward pointing accent, which indicated the potential change of pitch. A small dot represented no stress (Gimson, 1989, p. 229). The patterns for *examination* and *tobacco* would be

examination . • . ə .

tobacco . ə ₒ

(Differently sized squares (Allen, 1954) and circles (Bowen & Marks, 1992) fulfill the same function.)

J. Wells (1990, p. 683) separates the two types of secondary stress by designating the nonrhythmic secondary stress as tertiary and uses the subscript circle placed before the syllable to indicate it. Wells extends the usage of tertiary stress to the transcription of stress in phrases (p. 684); thus *fundamental* in the phrase *fundamental mistake* would have secondary stress on *fund-* /͵fʌnd/ and tertiary stress on *-ment-* /ˌment/, with primary stress on the first syllable of *mistake*. However, it is important to note that the stress pattern of *fundamental* in this phrase is different from its pattern in its citation form. When spoken in isolation, *fundamental* has primary stress on *-ment-* and secondary on *fund-*: /ˌfʌndə'mentᵊl/. Words of this pattern—secondary preceding primary—regularly shift their pattern when a primary stress occurs in a closely following word (as in *fundamental mistake*). Wells introduced the symbol ◀, a leftward pointing filled triangle, to indicate this stress shift. The following words illustrate Wells's transcription system:

academic	ˌækə'demiɪk ◀
	ˌacaˌdemic 'freedom
academician	əˌkædə'mɪʃᵊn
academicism	ˌækə'demɪˌsɪzəm
academy	ə'kædəmi

Four degrees of stress have regularly been acknowledged in American studies of English since Trager and Smith (1951):

primary / ' /
secondary /ᐱ/
tertiary / ` /
weak /ᵛ/

Simple words in citation form regularly use primary, tertiary, and weak stresses, such as *élevàtor* and *operàtor*; compound words often require a reduced primary stress, i.e. secondary, in the less prominent element, e.g. *élevàtor ôperàtor*.

In generative phonology (Chomsky & Halle, 1968, p. 16), a similar four stress system is acknowledged but symbolized by superscript numerals:

primary / [1] /
secondary / [2] /
tertiary / [3] /
quaternary/zero / [4] /

However, others in the generative tradition returned to accents, such as Durand (1990, p. 313):

primary / ´/
secondary / `/
tertiary / ˇ/
unstressed (no symbol)

The different uses of accents, particularly / ˋ / and / ˇ / for secondary and tertiary stresses has been highly confusing.

Finally, to return to iconic representations of stress, we have noted bold type in the case of Hawkins (1982). Brazil (1987) also used bold type for stressed ("protected") vowels, together with underlining, for the COBUILD dictionaries. Others have used capitals; italics have been used, and also italicized capitals (see Crystal, 1969, p. 161). O'Connor (1980) used the asterisk, but did not distinguish degrees of stress beyond stressed and unstressed. The advantage of an iconic representation is that phonetic prominence is matched by the visual, but its disadvantage is that degrees of prominence are not so easily captured.

The IPA set of symbols remains the most effective system for three degrees of stress; it is iconic in that the eye is drawn to a syllable by a mark; for primary stress, that mark is raised, for secondary stress it is low; syllables with less than secondary stress are deemed to be relatively unprominent and are thus not marked at all. If a tertiary degree of stress requires notation, then a low hollow circle, as in J. Wells (1990), is recommended.

IPA/Wells

1	primary	ˈba
2	secondary	ˌba
3	tertiary	˳ba
4	none	ba

Length

Length, as we noted, can affect both segments and syllables. In respect to segments, length of articulation is relevant to both consonants and vowels. Traditionally, the macron [ˉ] has been used to indicate distinctive vowel length, thus Latin:

agricola "farmer" (nominative)

agricolā "farmer" (ablative)

and English (*The Oxford English Dictionary*, 1933; *Concise Oxford Dictionary of Current English*, 1951; *Webster's Third New International Dictionary of the English Language*, 1961); a convention adopted also by *Webster's Third New International* (1961) to mark the length of r-less *bird*: bɜ̄d, subsequently adopted by Chomsky and Halle (1968, p. 51). As we have seen, the breve [ˇ] has traditionally indicated relative shortness as well as relative weakness.

However, the most common method of notation for length is the IPA symbol [ː]. Strictly speaking, it is not identical to the colon, as the points are triangular in shape, but as Pullum and Ladusaw (1986, p. 215) point out, the colon [:] is generally substituted as a more readily available typographical symbol.

The IPA symbol can readily be adapted to indicate degrees of length: half length by losing the lower point [ˈ] and extra length by doubling [::]. The half length symbol may indicate the clipped allophones of long vowels such as in English (Gimson, 1989, p. 97) or one unit in phonologically contrasting degrees of length as reported, for example, for Southern Mixe, Mexico (E.V. Pike, 1963, p. 55)

ˊpɛt   "a climb"

ˊpɛˈt   "broom"

ˊpɛːt   "Peter"

IPA retains the breve for "extra-short" vowels: [ă] and also typically the weaker element of a diphthong as in English *period*: ˈpɪ̆ŕĭəd.

A more obviously iconic symbol for length is the doubling of a symbol, which is more commonly used for the designation of relatively long consonants than of vowels. This is due to the interpretation of a typical case of long consonant over a syllable boundary. Thus, in English, the long consonants in *unknown* and *wholly*, /ʌnˈnəʊn/, /ˈhəʊlli/, can be interpreted as the coda and onset respectively of two syllables. These cases are more properly labeled "geminate" consonants to distinguish them from cases of contrastive consonant length within a syllable. Examples of the latter are reported, for instances of Shilh, Morocco (Westermann & Ward, 1933 p. 119):

bidd   "to stand still"

and of Luganda (Ladefoged, 1982, p. 226):

kulà   "grow up"

ˈkkulà   "treasure"

Symbol doubling has been used for representing long vowels, too, in Hausa for instance (Westermann & Ward, 1933:118):

babba   "big"

baabaa   "indigo"

lalle   "certainly"

laale   "welcome"

and English (McCarthy, 1952), see also Abercrombie (1964).

Rapidity of consonant articulation is captured in the design of IPA symbols for flaps and taps. The tap in American English *latter* and Spanish *pero* is, iconically, symbolized by a truncated form of the trill [r] symbol: [ɾ]. However this iconic truncation is not maintained by IPA for either the retroflex flap or the alveolar lateral flap.

Ladefoged reports in detail on a labiodental flap in Margi, Nigeria (Ladefoged, 1968, p. 18; 1982, pp. 154–155) but offers no symbol for it. E. V. Pike (1963, pp. 174–175) employed a raised wedge [ˇ] to represent all flap articulations, and identified the following: [f̌], [v̌], [ř], [*ř*] (i.e., voiceless), [ṛ̌] (i.e., retroflex), [ľ] and [ň]. A consistent use of a single diacritic has much to commend; see also Smalley (1963, p. 246). It must be distinguished from a subscript wedge [̬] used to indicate voicing in a consonant normally expected to be voiceless; J. Wells (1990, p. 703) uses the subscript wedge for the American tap in *latter*: [t̬] to designate its voicing rather than its tap articulation.

Length, it must be conceded, is not always recorded in transcription. Some linguists have chosen not to explicitly indicate the differences in length in English vowels, see Ward (1945) and Lewis (1972). The inherent length of a vowel is to be "understood" from the chosen vowel symbol without additional notation; thus /i/ in /bid/ *bead* is "understood" to be long; the length distinction between it and /ɪ/ is not explicitly transcribed.

A similar case of *understood* length appears in the description of syllable length in Japanese rhythm (Ladefoged, 1982, p. 226). A mora is a single unit of timing that consistently occupies a given length of time. In Japanese, the most common type of mora consists of a consonant followed by a vowel. A word such as [kakemono] ("scroll") contains four such morae. Another type of mora consists of a vowel alone; thus [iki] ("breath") contains two morae, each of which occupies the same length of time. A third type consists of a consonant alone; thus [nippoŋ] ("Japan") contains as many morae as [kakemono], namely [ni], [p], [po], and [ŋ]. The mora system is transparent in Japanese, as geminates, consonant clusters, and syllable-final consonants are not permitted. It follows that if the mora [i] and [ki] are the same length, the vowel [i] in the former is longer than [i] in the latter; this difference in length is *understood*, but it could be transcribed explicitly. The transcription [ii] is, in fact, two morae, not a single long vowel. Likewise the [p] of the mora [p] must be longer than the [p] within the mora [po]; the bilabial closure is held for the required length of time. But the extended closure is not normally marked.

These cases of nonmarking of length clearly indicate a phonological interpretation of the phonetic data.

Syllable Pitch

The kind of pitch accompanying the production of a syllable is relevant, as has been seen, in the determination of relative prominence, that is, stress, lexical tone in tone languages, and intonation. We shall consider intonation later, as with intonation, pitch is usually considered in the context of an utterance rather than in a single syllable or a sequence of syllables comprising a word.

Syllable pitch is usually described as either level or moving. K. L. Pike (1948) established the terms *register* and *contour* to describe relatively stable pitch in a syllable on the one hand and pitch movement on the other.

It is common to distinguish five levels in a register system: high, mid, low and intermediate levels, mid-high, and mid-low. In a contour system, it is necessary to distinguish (1) between directions of movement: falling, rising; (2) between degrees of movement: wide, narrow (a fall from high to low, as opposed to a fall from mid to low); and (3) options of movement: single, complex (a fall, as compared to a rapid sequence of fall and rise within a syllable).

The most common symbols used to designate pitch have been the acute, grave, and circumflex accents. However, these have been used for both register and contour pitches, and as has been discussed, for differing degrees of stress, too. Sweet (1877) used them solely for pitch movements, in iconic fashion:

  ´ = rising

  ` = falling

  ˘ = "compound" rising

and also

  ^ = "compound" falling

  – = level

Pike (1948, p. 50) recommended that when the accents were used in a contour system, they should precede the syllable:

  ˊba = high rising

  ˋba = high falling

  ˎba = low falling

  ⁻ba = high level

  _ba = low level, and so on

with the vertical position of the symbol indicating pitch height. In a register system, the accent would be placed above the syllable nucleus:

bá = high pitch

bà = low pitch

bā = mid pitch

An alternate symbol for mid pitch was a vertical stroke over the syllable nucleus: ba'. Lack of an accent could also play a significant role in the notation system.

However, when he indicated registers in Mazateco, Mexico (K. L. Pike 1948, p. 58) he resorted to superscript digits placed after the syllable: thus [1] = high, and [4] = low:

ya'ňchi[1]   "women"

nta'ti[2]   "kerosene"

nta'ʔa[3]   "saliva"

šo'hno[4]   "lime"

Ladefoged (1982, p. 229) also used digits, but 1 represented low pitch and 5 high.

In generative descriptions, it has been conventional to use H for high, M for mid, and L for low. In a two-feature system, high might be represented as +H and low as −H. Contours would be indicated as HL for fall, or HM if the fall was to mid only, and so on.

For Mandarin Chinese, Chao and Yang (1947) devised explicitly iconic "tone letters," with a horizontal or slanting stroke against a vertical line:

˥ = high level

˦ = mid to high rising

˯ = mid to low to mid high falling-rising

˩ = high to low falling

At this point, it should be noted that the term *tone* is generally used for phonological contrast and *pitch* for raw phonetic data. Thus, whereas Chao and Yang represent four "tone letters" for Mandarin Chinese, there are pitch variations for each of the four tones, in the same way as there are allophonic variations for each segmental phoneme. Within the range described earlier there are at least the following pitch levels and contours available.

	level	falling from high	from mid-high	from mid	from mid-low
high	˥				
mid-high	˦	˥˩			
mid	˧	˥˩	˦˩		
mid-low	˨	˥˩	˦˩	˧˩	
low	˩	˥˩	˦˩	˧˩	˨˩

rising from low	from mid low	from mid	from mid high
˩˥	˩˦	˩˧	˩˨
˩˦	˩˧	˩˨	
˩˧	˩˦		
˩˨			

falling-rising from high to high		from high to mid-high
˥˩˥		˥˩˦
˥˩˦		˥˩˧
˥˩˧		˥˩˨
˥˩˨		

and so on.

falling-rising from mid-high to high	falling-rising from mid-high to mid-high
˦˩˥	˦˩˦
˦˩˦	˦˩˧
˦˩˧	˦˩˨

and so on.

with similar falling-rising patterns starting from mid and mid-low, plus a similar range of falling-rising patterns starting from low, mid-low, mid, and mid-high and each terminating at either low, mid-low, mid and mid-high—an immense range.

None of the languages that employ pitch contrasts in words, the tone languages, remotely begin to exploit this full range. They all use between two and nine of these patterns as their basic "tonemes," while permitting a larger range of "allotones." The languages that primarily use level tones are known as register tone languages; those that exploit pitch movement are known as contour tone languages.

Finally, in this survey of the pitch notation, we refer to Westermann and Ward (1933) who employed a single iconic system of dots at differing heights to represent level tones and lines at different angles to represent contours. Thus in Ibo, Nigeria, is found:

isi [ˈ .]   smell

isi [ˈ ˈ]   head

isi [. \]   six

(Westermann & Ward, 1933, p. 135).

Finally, we return to the examples of a tone language that we considered at the beginning of this chapter. There are five separate, distinctive, tones in Thai; scholars have employed different notation means over the years to indicate them. It is also necessary to note slight variations in the phonetic detail of the description of the tones that represent genuine changes of pronunciation between the generations. Bradley, reported in K. L. Pike (1948, p. 21) and Henderson (1949) represent an older generation, which Leben (1980) also represents, while Lagefoged (1982) represents a younger generation. It is also worth noting that Gandour (1978, p. 43) suggests that Thai listeners readily distinguish all five tones in isolation; whatever changes take place, the five tone system is preserved.

	Bradley's description	Henderson's description and symbols	Leben's symbols	Ladefoged's description and symbols
1	middle	mid-level -kha "to dangle"	M	mid falling ⌍ 32
2	depressed	low level _kha "spice"	L	low falling ⌍ 21
3	falling	falling ˎkha "price"	HL	high falling ⌍ 51
4	circumflex	high rise- ^kha "to trade" fall (or acute)	H	high rising ⌐ 45
5	rising	rising kha "leg"	LH	low falling-rising ⌐ 215

Ladefoged's descriptions indicate much more clearly the contour quality of the tones of Thai. His tone letters are the most explicitly iconic; his numerical values (1 = low; 5 = high) give some detailed information but are less easy to interpret. Leben's symbols need the same kind of interpretation. Henderson's symbols are also iconic, but do not appear to be as accurate as Ladefoged's, note the extent of the fall and rise is not clearly given in items 3 and 5. A hint of the change in the phonetic shape of item 4 is given by Henderson's alternative label.

The IPA system of notation is given in Figure 6–1.

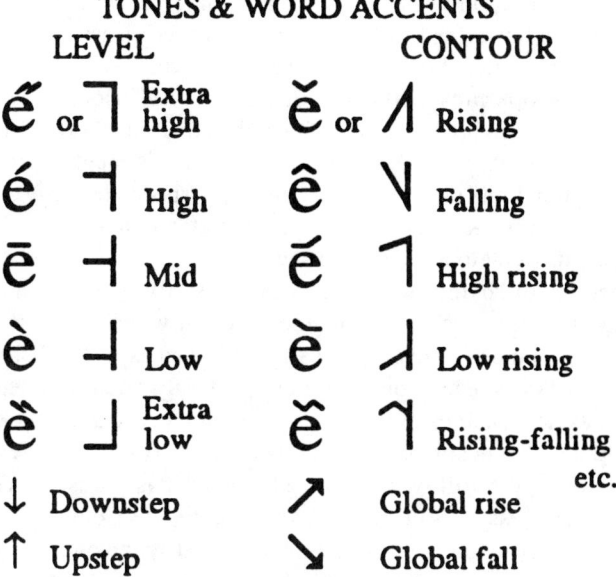

Figure 6-1. IPA System of Tone Notation. (With acknowledgments to the IPA.)

The "tone letters" are clearly the most explicit representation of both level and contour tones and are recommended for raw uninterpreted, phonetic transcription. The accents can be misleading—those of contour tones particularly so—unless K. L. Pike's convention is heeded: accents for level tones to be set above the syllable nucleus, accents for contour tones to be set before the syllable concerned. For phonologically interpreted data, a simple system of accents is probably the best recommendation.

Rhythm

Rhythm covers the characteristic combinations of more and less prominent syllables. There has been a controversy about the basis of the units of rhythm in English, and although differences of opinion on the nature of rhythmic units do not necessarily affect the design of notational symbols, they do affect the placement of symbols indicating rhythm unit boundaries.

Abercrombie's (1967) theory involves a rhythm unit, the foot, which by definition has always to begin with a prominent, stressed, syllable; consequently, any unstressed syllable follows a stressed one within the same foot. If any utterance begins with an unstressed syllable, a "silent stress" is assumed. The boundaries of the foot are assigned mechanically by the occurrences of accented syllables. This system operates without much difficulty in poetry and in what Halliday calls "rhythmic prose narrative" which is a "framework of a maximally regular rhythm" (Halliday, 1970, p. 120). However, it is much more difficult to identify such rhythm units in spontaneous, informal speech because of the hesitations, interruptions, revisions, and so on that characterize it. (Stress timing is also very much more difficult to recognize in such speech.)

Other theories of rhythm units are not necessarily based on meter, but on more detailed phonetic observations of the speed in which unstressed syllables are produced. O'Connor (1973) explains that utterances in English are broken into groups of syllables, each containing one and only one prominent, stressed, syllable. Unstressed syllables cluster around them. How can one tell if a given unstressed syllable that occurs somewhere between two stressed ones belongs to the preceding or to the following one? The answer is: "unstressed syllables which precede the stress are said particularly quickly" (O'Connor, 1973, p. 198), which leads one to assume that post-stress unstressed syllables are said relatively more slowly. That is the case in English: "In the group ‖ ɪt wəz *betə ‖ there are two unstressed syllables before the stress and one after it. The first two are said quickly, the last one not so quickly, taking the same amount of time as /be-/" (O'Connor, 1980, p. 97).

K. L. Pike (1962) gives more detail and is able to relate that detail to a wider range of languages. The junctural features of "stress-group rhythm waves," or rhythmic units, can be summarized in chart form (see Table 6–1).

The purpose of the chart is to aid the recognition of borders of feet by noting the more common features preceding or following a prominent (nucleus) syllable. It is the top row that is most relevant to English: Prenuclear unstressed syllables, those preceding the stressed syllable, are marked by a rapidly increasing level of loudness (crescendo), as well as by relative shortness as opposed to postnuclear unstressed syllables that are characterized by relative lengthening, lenis articulation (including devoicing), and decrescendo. All this means that for K. L. Pike, and O'Connor, units of rhythm do not necessarily *begin* with a stressed syllable; they must *contain* one but it may be preceded by unstressed syllables that are significantly characterized by a relative swiftness of articulation and crescendo.

Jassem and colleagues' description of rhythm units is broadly similar (see Jassem, Hill & Witten, 1984, pp. 206–208). They distinguish two kinds of rhythm units: "narrow rhythm units" in which the only or first syllable is accented and "total rhythm units," which include an anacrusis preceding the stressed syllable. An anacrusis consists of a syllable or a sequence of syllables, "which is characterized by being as short as possible," which is as short as is compatible with sufficiently distinct articulation of the constituent phones.

Table 6–1. Pike's Analysis of Rhythmic Units

Normal Rhythm Wave (= foot)		
	Prenucleus	**Nucleus**	**Postnucleus**
Frequent (often noncontrastive)	Crescendo (to) short	Loud (´to) Long (to:)	decrescendo (to) Long (to:) Lenis devoicing (tos) (toh)
Less frequent (often noncontrastive)		High pitch (to) Fortis contoids (tos)	Down glide (tò) Lenis contoids (tos) Glottal stop (to?)
Frequent (often contrastive)	Long vs. short High vs. low tone, etc.	Long vs. short High vs. low Ballistic vs. controlled	Long vs. short High vs. low tone etc. Ballistic vs. controlled

Jassem et al. thus concur with O'Connor's and Pike's observations on the distinctive significance of speed of articulation. They also noted that unstressed syllables following the nuclear, stressed syllable are roughly equal in length to the stressed syllable, itself, and are, therefore, significantly longer than the unstressed syllables preceding the stress. In other words, Jassem and colleagues assert that units in rhythm do not necessarily begin with a stressed syllable but may "accrue" with preceding unstressed syllables.

O'Connor, Pike and Jassem identify the borders of rhythm units on observable phonetic grounds, whereas Abercrombie (1967) and Halliday (1967) simply use the location of stressed syllables. The former seems right for both stress-timed rhythm such as that of English, and for syllable-timed rhythm, such as that of French. The latter seems to relate best to the style of speech associated with verse and "rhythmic prose narrative."

To indicate rhythmic unit boundaries, a variety of notational devices have again been employed. Abercrombie (1967) used the vertical bar [|], Halliday (1967) the slash [/]. K. L. Pike (1962) employed a low reverse slash [\ ] and O'Connor (1980) a word space, thus—taking account of different theories:

| which is the | train for | Crewe | please   (Abercrombie, 1967, p. 98)
/which is the /train for /Crewe /please   (Halliday)
'which\ is the 'train\ for 'Crewe\ 'please   (Pike)
'which isthe'train for'Crewe 'please   (O'Connor)

O'Connor's notation is the most explicitly iconic, but may be difficult to read. The choice of boundary mark may well depend on how the symbols are used in the transcription of intonation.

Intonation

It has been customary since Halliday (1967) to note three main systems within a description of intonation: *tonality*, the division of spoken discourse into discrete intonation units ("tone groups," "tone units" "breath groups," and "phonological phrases" are alternative terms); *tonicity*, the location of the most prominent pitch-bearing accent (known as the tonic or nucleus) within an intonation unit; and *tone*, the contrastive pitch movement or pitch level on the tonic syllable, and the pitch movement or pitch level in the preceding (pre-tonic) syllables. The term *accent* is used to refer to stressed syllables that could potentially bear changes of pitch discussed later. The term *tune* is often used to refer to the whole melody of an intonation unit, in other words, the sequence of pitch variations over all the accented and nonaccented syllables in the intonation unit combined.

Within the intonation unit, it has been customary since Palmer (1922) to note at least three parts to the structure of the unit: head, nucleus, and tail. Kingdon (1958) used the term *pre-head* to denote unstressed syllables before the first accented syllable (i.e. the head) and took the metaphor of head and tail further by using the term *body* to refer to stressed syllables that intervened between the first (the head) and the nucleus (or tonic). The structure of the tone group can be indicated as follows:

```
    A man is his own worst | enemy
                           |

   pretonic----------------> | tonic        (Halliday)
       |head -------------->  | *|tail      (Palmer)
    pre-|
   head|head --->|body----> | *|tail        (Kingdon)
   (* = nucleus)
```

Crystal (1969) identified the first accented syllable of the head as the "onset" syllable.

K. L. Pike (1947) established a different terminology. His theory of intonation proposed contrasting "primary contours" (= tunes), with a "beginning point" (= onset) on the first stressed syllable, an "ending point" containing a pitch glide (= tonic, nucleus), and a possible "direction-change point," in which the pitch changes from falling to rising or (rarely) rising to falling. Unstressed syllables preceding the beginning point of a contour are known as the "pre-contour" (= pre-head). Contours may also be "complex," such as an arrangement of two primary contours. There are other special contours that include chants, singsong, subsidiary contours, and so on.

A | man is his own worst | enemy

    | |

pre- | contour |

contour|beginning |ending

    |point | point   (Pike)

Linguists have differed on the number of significant tones, tunes and pitch levels in English (see Tench, 1990, pp. 398–440, for a full discussion). This is a matter of phonological interpretation, and the various alternatives are touched on in the discussion on notation.

Another factor frequently taken into account in intonation analysis is that of key. Sweet (1877, p. 96) described key as the general pitch of "each sentence, or sentence-group" and distinguished high, middle, and low: "Thus questions are naturally uttered in a higher key than answers, and parenthetic clauses in a lower key than those which state the main facts" (p. 96). Crystal (1969) also observed that stretches of utterances can be categorized as normal or at a lower or higher level than normal. However, Brazil (1975, 1978) identified high, mid, and low keys as independently meaningful choices, with mid key not to be considered as a speaker's normal pitch range, but as a meaningful option within a system.

Having made a preliminary sketch of the features that are relevant to the transcription of intonation, we turn first of all to the notation of tones and tunes. Sweet's (1877) form of notation was clearly iconic

level   –

rising   /

falling \

to which are added "compound tones":

compound rising ∨ (i.e., falling-rising)

compound falling ∧ (i.e., rising-falling)

Palmer (1922) added notations for heads that are also clearly iconic:

inferior head   ____

superior head   ═══

scandent head   /

He also distinguished high and low rises, again iconically, by vertical positioning of the accent:

    high rise   ´

    low rise   ,

O'Connor and Arnold (1961, 1973) introduced a similar distinction for high and low falls:

    high fall   `

    low fall   ˎ

Movements in the head extended Palmer's practice to identify further options in both the head and pre-head:

low head	A ˌman is his own worst —
high head	A 'man is his own worst —
falling head	A ˎman is his own worst —
rising head	A ˊman is his own worst —
low pre-head	_A man . . .
high pre-head	‾A man . . .

In the tail and body, high and low pitches are marked by a small circle at an appropriate height. A level tone is indicated by a sideways circumflex [>]. The scheme is displayed as follows:

    _A 'man is his °own °worst ˌenemy (O'Connor & Arnold)

Tench (1990) distinguished high and low varieties of falls and rises in addition to neutral forms, thus

    . . . `enemy . . . ˎenemy . . . ˌenemy

    . . . ´enemy . . . ˊenemy . . . ˌenemy

and high and low varieties of the complex tones, thus

    . . . ^enemy . . . ˄enemy

    . . . ˇenemy . . . ˅enemy

Glissando forms of the head are indicated by the presence of additional arrows, thus

A ⟍man is his ⟍own ⟍worst . . . .

A ⟋man is his ⟋own ⟋worst . . . .

(Glissando forms involve multiple pitch movements with the head, which are less prominent than the pitch movement on the nuclear-tonic syllable; they usually indicate a degree of forcefulness in speech.)

Palmer (1922), L.E. Armstrong & Ward (1926), and Crystal (1969) displayed tunes in visual form between parallel lines representing high and low, the so-called interlinear tonetic graph, commonly known as "tram lines." Larger dots represent accents, smaller dots other, unaccented syllables, and curves attached to the large dots (commonly known as "tadpoles") the pitch movements, thus:

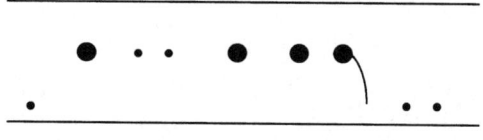

A man is his own worst en e my

Allen (1954) used a similar scheme, but with lines and dots:

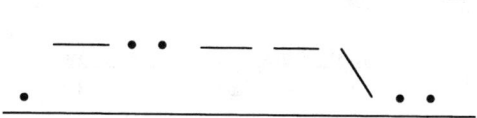

A man is his own worst en e my

A middle line was often included, so that five pitch levels could easily be identified. This is the display that Jones (1960) and Brown et al. (1980) use:

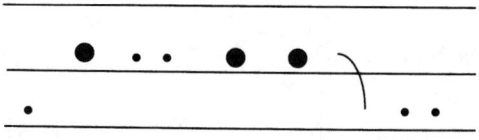

A man is his own worst en e my

K. L. Pike (1945) developed the continuous line display

A | man is his own worst e \nemy

Abercrombie (1967) and Ladefoged (1982) relied on a sketch representation of the tune:

A man is his own worst enemy

Bolinger (1986) displayed tones in such a way that the line of point followed a particular contour:

```
        man
              is his own worst e
    A                          n
                                 emy
```

K. L. Pike (1945) also described the intonation contours of American English in a four-pitch-level system, numbered 1 (high) to 4 (low). A pitch level was assigned to each stressed syllable, marked [°] and certain intermediate unstressed syllables, thus:

<u>A man is his own worst enemy</u>
°2–3 3–   °2–   °2–   °2–4

Armstrong and Ward (1926) presented a very simple numerical system: Tone 1 was falling; Tone 2 rising. Kingdon (1958) reversed this order: Tone I was rising, Tune II falling. O'Connor and Arnold (1973) listed 10 "tone groups," simply numbered 1 (low fall) to 10 (mid-level), in both unemphatic and emphatic forms. Halliday (1967) listed five primary tones:

Tone 1 (falling)   ‖\
Tone 2 (high rising)   ‖/
Tone 3 (low rising)   ‖/
Tone 4 (falling-rising)   ‖∨
Tone 5 (rising-falling)   ‖ᴧ

and a number of secondary tones in the tonic and the pre-tonic

Tone 1+ (wide)   ‖↑
Tone 1– (narrow)   ‖↳

Tone -1 (uneven) ˇ ˇ ˇ   ‖

Tone ...1 (listing) ‿ ‿ ‿   ‖

Tone 2 (falling-rising, pointed) ‖∨

Tone -2 (low)   ‒ ‒   ‖⁄

Tone -3 (low)   ‒ ‒   ‖∕

Tone 4 (low)   ‖˷

Tone 5 (low)   ‖˄

Bolinger (1989) listed a number of "profiles" by letters. Profile A has an abrupt fall; Profile B is marked by a jump up to the nuclear/tonic syllable, with any following unaccented syllables continuing with a gradual rise. Profile C has a drop down to the nuclear/tonic syllable and a small rise. Profile CA is "low-high-low," whereas Profile AC combines high fall and rise.

Profile A   — \

Profile B   — /

Profile C   — ∨

Profile CA   — ∧

Profile AC   — ∨

Profile CB is marked by a drop down to the nuclear/tonic syllable followed by a jump to high and a "slither"

Profile CB   — ⌒

Bolinger (1989, p. 4) comments, "The CB profile is rare in American English and Southern British, but is fairly common in other dialects and languages." (Scottish English could have been named here.)

A further classification of profies in sequence acknowledges higher and lower pitches, marked by acute and grave accents respectively

```
                     próm          héld
       héld                                    próm
I          him to his      i    I    him to his      i
                      s                           s
                      e.                          e.
```

are represented by A + Á and Á + A respectively, and

	ó		fóught them
fóught them			ó
We		We	
	f		f
	f.		f.

are represented by B + Á and B + Á. (Bolinger, 1989, p. 5)

Brazil (1975, 1978) also adopted letters to represent tones, but not an arbitrary set of letters simply listing them. Brazil distinguished primarily between falls and fall-rises, on the grounds that the former proclaim new information and the latter refer to common ground between speaker and hearer. Thus *p* stands for falls (*proclaiming*) and *r* for fall-rises (*referring*). Therefore, *p+* is a rise-fall, meaning that the information is also new for the speaker; *r+* is a rise and represents the speaker's "intervention" in the sense of taking a positive initiative in invoking common ground, such as asking a question. *o* represents "oblique orientation," such as a speaker, or quite typically a reader reading text aloud, does not engage in any of the above roles; phonetically, *o* is realized as a mid level tone. Thus

   p A MAN is his own worst E̲nemy

Crystal (1969, pp. 144–148) introduced a further refinement in the notation of step-downs and step-ups within the head. He noted two degrees of step-down (or "drop"), indicated by long or short vertical arrows, three degrees of step-ups (or "boosters"), and pitch continuance, indicated by a horizontal arrow. An example of this is given in Figure 6–2. Although the full system was used in Crystal & Davy (1969), it was simplified to a single degree of step-up [↑] in Crystal and Davy (1975).

Crystal also identified the onset syllable distinctively, with a vertical bar [|]. The onset syllable is the initial accented syllable in the head; the identification of it is important, as shall be seen, in the key system, although Crystal, himself, did not explore that function. Subsequent stressed syllables between the onset and tonic syllables were marked with the simple stress mark unless there was significant step up or down, as indicated above. Thus:

   a | man is his ↑ own 'worst È̲Nemy

Brazil (1975, 1978) indicated the onset by capitals, without underlining, (underlining indicated the nuclear-tonic syllable).

In generative treatments of intonation, the onset syllable was marked as the initial boundary of the contour. Their formula often took the form of a series of three references: the onset syllable, the initial point of pitch height of the tonic, and the end, or terminal, point of pitch height, see Liberman (1979). Thus:

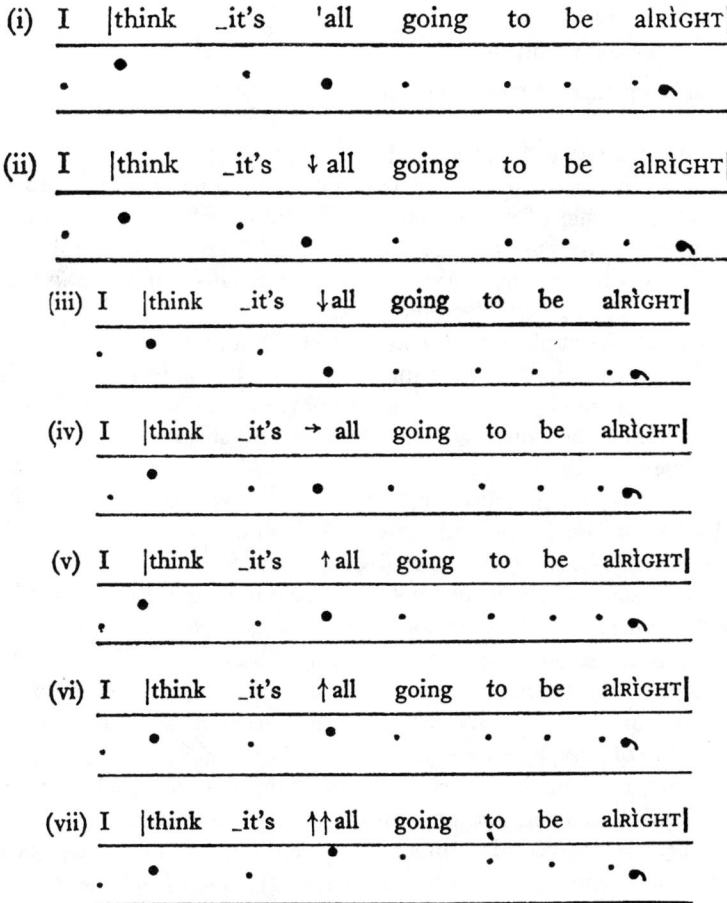

Figure 6–2. An example of Crystal's notation system. (Crystal 1969, 145–146)

A man is his own worst enemy

```
man         enemy
 |          |    |
L-M        H-M   L
```

Different contours representing the "lexicon" of intonation were recorded with such strings of letters:

L-M H-M L was unmarked

L H L represented surprise

L H-H L represented tempered surprise

etc. (See Tench, 1990, p. 437, for a full table.)

The notation of tonic (or nuclear) syllables within intonation units follows a similar pattern to that of stress. As stress is the manifestation of prominence within a word or rhythm unit, the tonic syllable is the most prominent stress amongst a sequence of rhythm units. The same range of symbols has been employed for both stress and the tonic syllable.

Palmer (1922) employed vertical strokes for nonnuclear stressed syllables and reserved accent marks for the tonic syllable. O'Connor and Arnold (1961) followed the same policy; although they employed a wider range of symbols for stressed syllables, they distinguished the tonic by an exclusive use of accent marks (see previous discussion).

Allen (1954) indicated the tonic by bold type, Halliday (1967) and Brazil (1975, 1978) by underlining, and Crystal (1969) (see previous), Brown (1990), Gussenhoven (1984), and many others by capitals.

American studies have tended not to indicate the tonic because of the prevalence of the concept of whole contours; the tonic is usually identifiable from the pitch direction change point (see previous examples from Pike and from Liberman).

The highly visual schemes employing dots and curves within "tramlines" rely primarily on dots with tails (the "tadpoles") to indicate the tonic in addition to the direction of pitch (see above).

The notation of the boundaries of intonation units must take into account decisions taken elsewhere on the notation of rhythm units and pauses. As we noted, K. L. Pike (1945) differentiated between two types of pause because of their function at borders of contours or pause groups: [l] indicated a tentative pause, [l l] indicated a final pause, which was usually of greater duration. These symbols effectively marked the boundaries of intonation units. O'Connor (1980) employs the same symbols for apparently similar purposes.

Halliday (1967) used a single slash [/] to indicate the borders of rhythm units and a double slash [//] for intonation unit borders. Brazil (1975, 1978) also used a double slash for the latter purpose, whereas Clark and Yallop (1990) used a double bar [l l].

Crystal (1969) used a single, thin, bar [l] to indicate the onset syllable, and used a single, bold, bar [ ] for borders.

Many studies have concentrated on single utterances and, consequently, the marking of borders has been irrelevant.

Tench (1988, 1990) placed each intonation unit on a separate line and thus required no special symbol to mark the borders.

Finally, a number of devices have been employed to indicate key. Sweet (1877) invented the following symbols:

```
high      ⌈
middle    ⌈ L
low       L
```

and commented: "The middle key may also be left unmarked" (p. 96).

Key plays an important role in Brazil's (1975) description of intonation and thus is explicitly indicated. This is done by the height of a line of text. *H, M, L* appear on the left margin in a vertical display, with lines of text appearing at the appropriate height, e.g.

H   FIRST   *r*+ if we <u>can</u>
M p <u>WELL</u> // *o*   LET'S // *p* a<u>GREE</u> //   // *r*+ mister <u>SCOTT</u>
L

(from Brazil, Coulthard, & Jones, 1980, p. 182)

Cruttenden (1986) indicated change of key by a double slash, in contrast to single slashes for intonation unit boundaries:

> Well I saw `Jim the other ˏday // inci`dentally / he's just got `married again // and ˇhe said . . . (Cruttenden, 1986, p. 129)

Miller and Tench (1982) resorted to a series of vertical arrows at the beginning of an intonation unit to indicate the level of key. Five normal levels were postulated: The highest was indicated by a double arrow pointing upwards, with descending levels indicated by, respectively, a single arrow, no arrow, and a single, or double, arrow pointing downwards. Exclamations that were deemed to be higher than high key were indicated by a triple upwards pointing arrow.

With regard to the identification of intonational components in speech, some investigators have noted that it is not always possible to identify tone groups and nuclei following traditional criteria. For example, the definitions of tone groups and nuclear tones that have been advanced by Halliday (1967) and Crystal (1969), have been strongly contested by Brown et al. (1980) for Edinburgh English, and Rahilly (1991) for Belfast English. The evidence provided by these studies suggests that it may be profitable to adopt a less phonetically rigid approach to identifying intonational components, especially for disordered speech.

Articulatory and Phonatory Settings and Paralinguistic Features

Finally, we turn to a number of features that characterize an individual's speech in utterances or part utterances. Some of these features were touched upon in *Voice Quality* above (p. 109f); a fuller description appears in Crystal and Davy

(1969) and Laver (1980). A distinction can be made between voice qualities proper and articulatory settings—the former relate to types of phonation and the latter to distinctive configurations in the supralaryngeal cavities.

Laver (1980, p. 45) identified the following lingual articulatory settings, shown in Figure 6–3 and he suggested symbols and diacritics for the notation of each.

In addition, Laver identified: tip articulation, blade articulation, and retroflex articulation; together with the following labial articulatory settings: labiodentalization, open rounding, close rounding, spread lips; also nasalization and de-nasalization, vertical movements of the larynx and jaw positions. A complete and revised set of symbols for these voice qualities (Ball, Esling, & Dickson, 1994) is presented in Figure 6–4 and is also included in the Appendix.

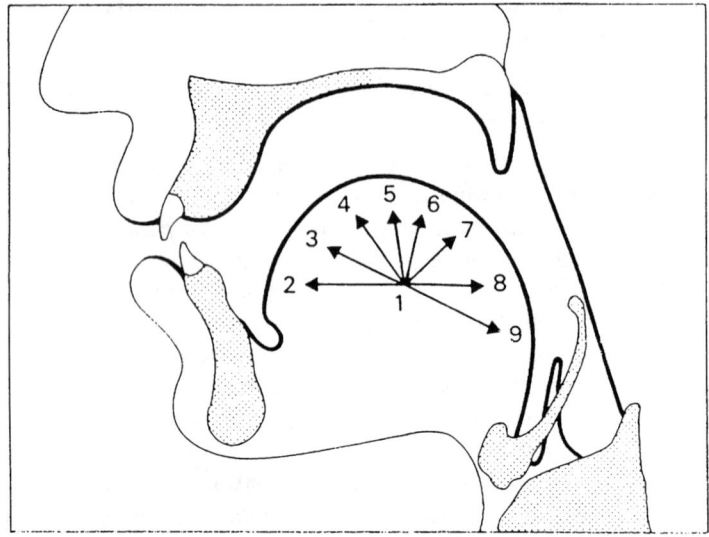

Sagittal section of the vocal tract in the neutral setting, showing radial directions of movement of the centre of mass of the body of the tongue in lingual settings

1. Centre of mass of the tongue
2. Dentalization
3. Alveolarization
4. Palato-alveolarization
5. Palatalization
6. Velarization
7. Uvularization
8. Pharyngalization
9. Laryngo-pharyngalization

Figure 6–3. Articulatory settings for voice quality. (Reprinted with permission of Cambridge University Press.)

VoQS: Voice Quality Symbols

AIRSTREAM TYPES

Œ	oesophageal speech	Ю	electrolarynx speech
Ю	tracheo-oesophageal speech	↓	pulmonic ingressive speech

PHONATION TYPES

V	modal voice	F	falsetto
W	whisper	C	creak
V̰	whispery voice (murmur)	V̰	creaky voice
V̤	breathy voice	Ç	whispery creak
V!	harsh voice	V!!	ventricular phonation
V̰!!	diplophonia	V̰!!	whispery ventricular phon.
V̪	anterior or pressed phonation	W̱	posterior whisper

SUPRALARYNGEAL SETTINGS

L̝	raised larynx	L̞	lowered larynx
Vᶦ	labialized voice (open round)	Vʷ	labialized voice (close round)
V̈	spread-lip voice	Vᵛ	labio-dentalized voice
V̺	linguo-apicalized voice	V̻	linguo-laminalized voice
V˞	retroflex voice	V̪	dentalized voice
V̳	alveolarized voice	V̡ʲ	palatoalveolarized voice
Vʲ	palatalized voice	Vˠ	velarized voice
Vʁ	uvularized voice	Vˤ	pharyngealized voice
V̰ˤ	laryngo-pharyngealized voice	Vᴴ	faucalized voice
Ṽ	nasalized voice	V̾	denasalized voice
J̞	open jaw voice	J̝	close jaw voice
J̰	right offset jaw voice	J̠	left offset jaw voice
J̟	protruded jaw voice	Θ	protruded tongue voice

USE OF LABELED BRACES & NUMERALS TO MARK STRETCHES OF
SPEECH AND DEGREES AND COMBINATIONS OF VOICE QUALITY

[ˈðɪs ɪz ˈnɔ·məl ˈvɔɪs {3V! ˈðɪs ɪz ˈveri ˈhɑ·ʃ ˈvɔɪs 3V!} ˈðɪs ɪz ˈnɔ·məl ˈvɔɪs
wʌns ˈmɔ· {L̝1V! ˈðɪs ɪz ˈles ˈhɑ·ʃ ˈvɔɪs wɪð ˈloʊəd ˈlæɹɪŋks 1V!L̝}]

© 1994 Martin J. Ball, John Esling, Craig Dickson

Figure 6–4. VoQS Chart. (With acknowledgments to ICPLA.)

Degrees of muscular tension can also be noted. Duckworth et al. (1990) reintroduced diacritics for fortis and lenis articulation of segments. The following symbols may be used for denoting general muscular settings:

tense articulation	{V̬}
lax articulation	{V̜}

Finally, Crystal and Davy (1969) identified the following other paralinguistic features in their investigations:

1. Variations in tempo, marked as follows:

   allegro   {alleg}

   allegrissimo   {allegriss}

   lento   {lento}

   lentissimo   {lentiss}

   accelerando   {accel}

   rallentando   {rall}

2. Variations in volume:

   forte   {f}

   fortissimo   {ff}

   piano   {p}

   pianissimo   {pp}

   crescendo   {cresc}

   diminuendo   {dimin}

3. Variations in rhythmicality:

   rhythmic   {rhythm}

   arhythmic   {arhythm}

   staccato   {stac}

   legato   {leg}

4. Various vocal effects, simultaneous with speech, which inevitably have an effect on the overall quality of speech. These would be simply labeled within the braces, as in:

   {laughter}

   {sobbing}

   {tremulousness}, and so on.

Transcribing Disordered Prosody

For most of this book, we have concentrated on the description and transcription of individual sounds of speech, such as segmental features. This concentration reflects a general tendency in studies of disordered speech to highlight segmental abnormalities, with rather rather little attention being paid to suprasegmental aspects of speech such as intonation, rhythm, and loudness, for example (the neglect of suprasegmental approaches to clinical speech analysis is discussed further in Brewster, 1989). Chapter 6, however, suggested that a purely segmental transcription of speech is essentially limited, because it fails to take account of aspects of speech that have important linguistic and paralinguistic effects. That chapter established the need to record suprasegmental or prosodic aspects of speech in transcription and provided explanations of suprasegmental phenomena, such as voice quality, stress, length, pitch and intonation. It also showed that suprasegmental aspects operate over syllables, rather than at the level of individual consonants or vowels. In this chapter, we look at how speech pathologists can perform suprasegmental transcription in the clinical context and discuss the value of such a transcription. Following the structure of Chapter 6, we will look at the transcription of voice quality, length, stress, pitch, and intonation, in turn, and also broaden the scope of suprasegmental elements to look briefly at intensity and speech rate in disordered speech. (These are not discussed in Chapter 6, because transcriptions of normal speech seldom need to record differing degrees of vocal intensity or of speech rate.)

The Value of Suprasegmental Transcription in the Clinic

In the clinical context, speech pathologists encounter a wide range of abnormalities resulting from disturbances to the segmental or suprasegmental aspects of speech; many disorders may well combine segmental *and* suprasegmental disturbances. We have indicated in Chapter 2 that segmental breakdown has consequences for the intelligibility of speech. If, for example, a speaker fails to produce the phonemic contrasts that are characteristic of the native language, listeners are likely to have difficulty processing the message. The breakdown or impairment of the suprasegmental system is also likely to interfere with normal communication. For instance, with particular reference to intonation, one function of the nuclear tone in a stretch of speech is to draw the listener's attention to new pieces of information in the discourse (see Halliday, 1970).[1] In disordered speech, however, it may be that speakers consistently give nuclear prominence to pieces of information that are not new. In the utterance given as example 1a following, for instance, the nuclear tone (indicated by upper case letters) is located on *town*. Once *town* has been established in the discourse, it no longer requires highlighting in the form of nuclear prominence, and one might envisage a normal utterance proceeding along the lines of 1b, in which the nucleus is located on the next new piece of information, such as *nice*. Disordered speakers may not, however, follow the general pattern whereby nuclear prominence correlates with new information. An example of this is given in 1c, in which the nucleus remains on *town*. If speakers locate the nuclear tone on an item in the utterance that does not correlate with new information, then they may be misunderstood by listeners, whose attention is drawn to inappropriate items.

(1a) We went to the TOWN.

(1b) It wasn't a very NICE town.

(1c) It wasn't a very nice TOWN.

A second example of the effect of suprasegmental impairment relates to pitch. It is known from the literature that F_0 carries emotional and psychological information in speech (see, for example, Abberton et al., 1985; Cutler, 1980; Kramer, 1963; Rosen, Fourcin & Moore, 1981). It has been shown that happiness and joy, for example, correlate with high pitch level, wide pitch range, and a high degree

---

[1]This correlation between the nuclear tone and new information is a general tendency in normal speech. There are, of course, examples of nuclear prominence occurring on already-mentioned items, see Knowles, 1987.

of pitch variability. Boredom, by contrast, correlates with low pitch level, narrow range, and comparatively small pitch variability. Abnormalities in the F_0 contour are therefore often used as an index to psychological disorders in a number of studies. For example, Leff and Abberton (1981) found that monotonous voice (which the authors define as narrowing in the normal range of variation in pitch) in schizophrenic patients correlated with damping of emotion and that narrowing of pitch range was common among patients with a severe degree of depression (see also Nilsonne, Sundberg, Ternstrom, & Askenfelt, 1988). It may, therefore be the case that restricted pitch movement among disordered speakers creates the impression that the speakers are lacking in positive personality traits. On the other hand, an excessively wide pitch range may also convey misinformation concerning the speaker's personality. The effect of pitch characteristics of speech on listeners' assessment is summarized:

> Either an abnormally restricted or extended pitch range may be responsible for uncomfortable misunderstandings of the speaker's attitude, the former tending to give an impression of lack of interest or depression while the latter . . . often sounds much more aggressive than the speaker intends. (Parker 1983, p. 242)

We have indicated that the transcription of disordered prosody is an area that requires attention among speech clinicians to enhance patients' communicative skills both on a linguistic and a paralinguistic level. In the clinical literature, however, there is some vagueness concerning exactly what constitutes suprasegmentals and how prosodic phenomena ought to be transcribed (this vagueness is discussed in Crystal, 1985). This chapter attempts to clarify the situation by suggesting ways in which clinicians can embark on suprasegmental transcription and by identifying the key areas that are likely to be affected in a range of speech disorders. Where feasible, we present the IPA conventions for transcribing suprasegmentals in normal speech that can also be used to capture suprasegmental features in disordered speech. We also highlight the suprasegmental elements of extIPA, the recent developments of the IPA that are explicitly intended for the transcription of disordered speech (the extIPA conventions for transcribing segmental aspects of speech are discussed in detail in Chapter 5). In addition, we pinpoint some of the areas that cannot be captured by either of these resources and make suggestions for their symbolization.

Voice Quality

In Chapter 6, it was stated that the term voice quality may refer to phonatory setting and to supra-glottal articulatory setting and it was shown that voice quality settings can operate at the level of individual segments or over a succession of segments. For the purposes of suprasegmental transcription, we are required to indicate voice quality deriving form both phonatory and supra-glottal settings and at the level of stretches of speech. ExtIPA has adopted many of Laver's (1980) influential descriptions of voice quality and offers symbols for both kinds of setting.

ExtIPA recognizes five phonatory settings, breathy/whispery, whisper, creak, ventricular or harsh voice, and falsetto. They are marked in transcription using braces to indicate the stretch of speech affected, following the pattern for marking speech rate and intensity, as follows:

[xxx {V̰ xxxx V̰} xxx]	breathy/whispery
[xxx {V̬ xxxx V̬} xxx]	whisper
[xxx {V̰ xxxx V̰} xxx]	creak
[xxx {V!! xxxx V!!} xxx]	ventricular voice
[xxx {F xxxx F} xxx]	falsetto

In the case of supra-glottal settings, the IPA scheme for marking secondary articulations is adequate for transcribing disordered speech. This uses superscript symbols to mark labialized, labio-dentalized, palatalized, velarized, and pharyn-gealized voice qualities. The use of these diacritics is illustrated below:

[xxx {Vʷ xxxx Vʷ} xxx]	labialized
[xxx {Vᵛ xxxx Vᵛ} xxx]	labio-dentalized
[xxx {Vʲ xxxx Vʲ} xxx]	palatalized
[xxx {Vˠ xxxx Vˠ} xxx]	velarized
[xxx {Vˤ xxxx Vˤ} xxx]	pharyngealized
[xxx {Ṽ xxxx Ṽ} xxx]	nasalized

These diacritics can, of course, accompany individual segments as appropriate, as illustrated in example 2:

(2) [ð\ð:ə {V̰ ə\ə\ə V̰} ˈhwɔɪld]

For detailed investigation in the area of voice quality, it is likely that clinicians will require access to a wider set of symbols for transcribing voice quality settings than those given above. An extensive set is provided by VoQS: Voice Quality Symbols (Ball, Esling, & Dickson, 1994, see also Chapter 6). This set will be included in the forthcoming tutorial program for transcribing disordered spech and voice qualities (to be produced by Kay Elemetrics).

An additional point of interest in the transcription of voice quality is the direction of air-flow during phonation. In normal speakers, the airstream is usually pulmonic egressive. Among disordered speakers, however, a pulmonic ingressive airstream may operate. ExtIPA uses a downward arrow to indicate this type of airstream in single segments such as [s↓], for example, or over longer stretches of speech, as in:

[dɪfɹənt sɛn ↓}təɹz↓}ɪn speən]

Stress

We define stress here as phonetic exaggeration, following Laver's (1994) explanation of the term:

> Where one of two otherwise identical syllables is made more prominent than the other by an exaggeration of the value of one or more of the phonetic parameters of pitch, loudness, duration or quality . . . the more prominent syllable can be said to receive more stress. (p. 511)

As demonstrated in Chapter 6, the IPA offers two symbols for marking syllabic stress or exaggeration, that is ['], for main stress and [ˌ] for secondary stress,[2] as illustrated in the words in example 3 below:

(3) sic transit gloria mundi

[ˌsɪk 'trænzɪt ˌgloːriə 'mʊndi]

In disordered speech, we posit three main problems with stress organization: Speakers may use excessive amounts of stress, they may omit it completely, or they may use it inappropriately by locating it on the wrong syllable in the word. The IPA provides the means for recording all of these abnormalities. Excessive stress can be indicated by double or triple stress marks, as in ["] or ["'], respectively, placed before the relevant syllable.

Also relevant to stress may be the features of "stronger and weaker articulation" suggested by extIPA. The notions of stronger and weaker articulation relate to the general physiological force with which a syllable is produced. In the case of disordered speech, it may be that speakers employ either more or less physiological force than is normal for a production and the effect may be that the speech is perceived as being either over- or understressed. The IPA extensions offer two new diacritics to cover the strength of articulation feature [‖] for strong and [ˌ] for

---

[2]Secondary stress, according to Clark and Yallop (1995, p. 298) represents an "intermediate" degree of stress, between primary and zero stress. They say: "A syllable containing any other vowel quality [than schwa] but not given prominence by the normal devices of English stress marking, will then count as having secondary stress." Examples are the final syllable in *pedigree* and *indicate*.

weak, with both diacritics placed under the respective segment symbol. Example 4 (taken from Ball, Code, Rahilly, & Hazlett, 1994, p. 74) demonstrates the diacritic for strong articulation (in this example, the backslash marks the boundary between rapidly reiterated parts of the utterance, see below):

(4) [ð:e wɪl ɪnv\ẙɔːlv]

It is clear from the above example that both stress and strength of articulation are often marked on the same syllable.

The patterning of stressed and unstressed syllables in speech contributes to the overall rhythm of the speech. Clearly, if stress is omitted, overemphasized, or inappropriately distributed this has consequences for the overall rhythmic structure of the speech. If, for example, every syllable receives the same degree of stressing, the speech will sound labored and placement of stress on unusual syllables may render it disjointed. For example, W. Wells' (1994) study of a child suffering from a severe developmental speech disorder shows that the stress patterning in the child's speech leads to a slow, staccato rhythm which gives an impression of disjointedness.

To arrive at a comprehensive assessment of the rhythmic structure of a patient's speech, therefore, we must include stress marking in transcription.

Length

Length refers to the duration of a segment or syllable in time. As has been noted in Chapter 6, length is often seen as a property of individual vowels and consonants. Nevertheless, Ball (1993, pp. 92–93) has pointed out that length on one phonetic segment affects the adjacent segment. For example, if a syllable has a long vowel, it will have a short consonant and, if the vowel is short, the consonant will be longer. Length therefore, is not restricted to individual segments, but operates over larger domains. In this sense, it can be considered as suprasegmental.

In the case of disordered speech, abnormal length may occur in two main contexts, within syllables and in pauses. In syllables, for example, speakers may shorten or lengthen syllables in particular contexts so that they become excessively short or excessively long compared with those in normal speech. The IPA has two diacritics for marking long segments, [ː] for fully long and [ˈ] for half long, and one diacritic to mark short segments, i.e., [˘]. If one wishes to record segments that are extra long or extra short in disordered speech, repetitions of these marks, [ːː] for extra-long, and [˜] for extra short can be used.

The second abnormality in terms of length that may occur in disordered speech relates to unfilled pauses. Pauses may be excessively long or they may be located in unusual places in the utterance compared to normal speech. In fact, our judgment of whether pause length is normal or not relies on impressionistic assessments of its length in relation to the overall tempo and rhythm of an utterance, rather than on any standardized measurements in seconds. This is because a long pause in one speaker's production may well be shorter than a short pause in another's (see Quirk, Duckworth, Svartvik, Rusiecki, & Colin, 1964 for a discussion of pause length relative to overall speed of speech). Descriptions of pause length, therefore, tend to be relativistic, rather than based on absolute measurements, along the lines of "very short pause," and a "pause equal to one beat of the speaker's rhythm" (see Fawcett & Perkins, 1980, for example).

The recent revision of extIPA offers a three-way distinction for marking unfilled pauses, short pause, medium-length pause and long pause. The pauses are represented by one, two, or three dots, respectively, enclosed within rounded brackets, as illustrated in example 5:

(5) ['lastɪn ˌoʊvəɹ 'fɔɹ 'wiks (..) 'hɛld ə ʔat 'f\fɔɹtin (…)]

It has been noted (Ball, Code, Rahilly, & Hazlett, 1994) that this three-way distinction may not always be adequate for reflecting abnormal pause length. This may be the case, for example, if there is an excessively long pause lasting for several seconds at a particular point in an utterance. In this case, we suggest that the pause should be transcribed by indicating its time length within the parentheses, e.g., [xxxxx (5 sec) xxxxx]. In the light of our comments above that assessments of suprasegmental normality are made relative to each individual's own tempo and rhythm, we do not wish to suggest that absolute pause length is a suitable measure of normality among speakers. A specified pause length in a transcription is to be taken merely as an indication that the pause is excessively long for that particular speaker.

One further feature of disordered speech may be responsible for interfering with the length of syllables, reiteration. Reiteration is the repetition of segments, syllables or longer stretches of speech. It occurs principally in stuttered speech and is listed in extIPA within the category of manner of articulation. Clearly, if a segment in a syllable is reiterated, the reiteration will result in a longer than usual syllable and in this sense, reiteration relates to suprasegmental length. To transcribe reiteration, extIPA recommends that the back slash is used to separate rapidly reiterated parts of an utterance from one another, as in example 6.

(6) [ðə s\s\s\s emi faɪnəlz]

Length is inextricably linked with stress and rhythm. In the section on stress above, we defined stressed syllables as those that are phonetically exaggerated in some way. Our perception of stress may derive from phonetic exaggeration in terms of syllable pitch or loudness, for example, or it may be a result of a combination of exaggeration in a range of phonetic parameters. In particular, syllables are often identified as stressed because they are phonetically lengthened. Length is, therefore, an important contributor to the rhythmic framework of an utterance and needs to be recorded in transcription.

Pitch and Intonation

Although we have chosen to discuss pitch and intonation under the same heading, one should be aware that they are not synonymous terms. Pitch refers specifically to the fundamental frequency (F_0) of the voice, its height and variability. Intonation, on the other hand, is the systematic harnessing of pitch patterns to convey meaning on a number of levels. For example, the pitch shape of individual tones may convey sentence type and the pitch height may convey conversational turn completion or incompletion and clausal relationships (see Rahilly, 1991; Tench, 1988). In one sense, then, the pitch/intonation division parallels the phonetic/phonological division described in Chapter 2. Pitch is the raw, phonetic material and intonation is a meaningful, phonological system within the language.

In the past, few investigators have attempted to devise transcriptional conventions for representing pitch and intonation in disordered speech. Most research attention has been devoted to pitch and to pitch height in particular, but pitch characteristics are not usually recorded in transcription. Although several studies have presented analyses of pitch deviation in pathological speech (see for example Leder et al., 1987; Leff & Abberton, 1981; Nilsonne, Sundberg, Ternstrom, & Askenfelt, 1988), the findings have no direct application to the transcription of pitch characteristics.

For the transcription of intonation, the IPA offers diacritical tone marks to indicate the pitch height and pitch direction of tones (see Chapter 6). We suggest, however, that these tone marks are problematic for the transcription of intonation in both normal and disordered speech. There are two main difficulties. First, the tone marks may pose problems for interpretation. For example, the IPA suggests that high rises should be transcribed as [˦] or [ˊ]. In traditional systems of tonetic stress marking, dating back to Kingdon (1958), however, high rises are transcribed by a single symbol, that is [ˊ]. The IPA's use of [ˆ] for simple falls and [ˇ] for simple rises presents further difficulties. Most transcribers use these symbols to indicate rise-falls and fall-rises respectively (see Altenberg, 1987; Cruttenden, 1986; Knowles, 1986). There is, of course, some experimental evidence to suggest that rising tones may be preceded by a short falling onset or falling tones by a brief rising onset (see Ainsworth & Lindsay, 1984, 1986), but the inclusion of this kind information in transcription seems unnecessarily cumbersome and may lead to ambiguity in the interpretation of tone marks. A similar situation exists for IPA transcriptions of complex tones, rise-falls and fall-rises.

It offers [~] and [ꜛ] as alternative transcriptions for rise-falls, for example. Again, the transcription of an initial falling onset in a rise-fall is to be transcribed, as is suggested by the first alternative, the symbol may be difficult to interpret. These potential problem areas could be avoided by retaining the traditional tonetic stress mark system following Kingdon (1958). These are given below:

High Fall (`)	Low Fall (ˎ)
High Rise (´)	Low Rise (ˏ)
High Fall-Rise (ˇ)	Low Fall-Rise (ˬ)
High Rise-Fall (^)	Low Rise-Fall (˄)
High Level (¯)	Low Level (_)

The second source of difficulty with the IPA conventions for transcribing intonation is that they operate with a nuclear tone based approach. The motivation for this approach seems to be that the nucleus is the central element from which the entire tone-unit shape is thought to be predictable (this is suggested, for example, in Halliday, 1970). We suggest, however, that nuclear tone-based analyses are essentially limited, because they examine a relatively small number of syllables in any given sample and neglect potentially important intonational variation extending over longer stretches of speech. If we assume that intonational abnormality is limited to the nucleus and, as a consequence, fail to examine the other elements within the tone-unit, our analysis is likely to be seriously flawed.

Most investigators of American English intonation (emanating from K. L. Pike, 1945) have attempted to look at whole intonation contours, rather than individual nuclei as British investigators have done. They have, therefore, examined intonation on a more global level and have identified what essentially amount to tune shapes or configurations of pitch contours that correlate with attitudinal stances such as surprise (Sag & Liberman, 1975) and warning (Liberman, 1975), for example. Nevertheless, American analysts still highlight the role of the nucleus in determining the configuration. Although some British analysts have also investigated tune shape, they also suggest that the shape is predictable from the nucleus shape alone (see Halliday, 1970, for example). However, we have some evidence to show that the full range of intonation abnormalities that may occur in disordered speech cannot be captured by using a nuclear tone based method. For example, a study of postlingual deaf speakers (Rahilly, 1991) has demonstrated that intonational abnormalities can occur in a wide of intonational components.

To facilitate an open-ended approach to intonation analysis so we can capture the potential range of abnormalities that may occur in disordered speech, we recommend the use of interlinear transcription as a tool. The method of recording intonation patterns in interlinear transcription was described in Chapter 6. Briefly, so-called "tram lines" represent the upper and lower limits of a speaker's pitch range. Within those lines, tone marks are placed in sections that represent the general area of the pitch range in which a syllable was uttered, and the shape of the syllable.

The model of intonation analysis we use here, however, is somewhat different from those described in Chapter 6 for normal speech. This is because it may be inappropriate to use the same criteria for identifying intonational units in normal and disordered speech. For example, one standard definition of a nucleus equates it with the syllable that contains the maximum amount of pitch movement in the tone unit (see Crystal 1969). It may, however, be impossible to find such a syllable in disordered speech and it may be that other intonational elements are not characterized by the same phonetic criteria that operate in normal intonation. We therefore suggest an alternative model of intonational analysis which avoids the specific associations of existing descriptions. The elements of the present model are presented and defined in Figure 7–1. The central elements are the **tone sequence**, the **prominence** or **prominences**, the **leading syllable** and **leading segment**, and the **final segment**.

At this point, we provide a brief demonstration of how we might apply the above model of intonation analysis to one variety of disordered speech, postlingual deafness. It has been shown (Rahilly, 1991) that there is a tendency for speakers who are postlingually deaf to produce stretches of speech that contain rather little or no pitch movement at all. Interlinear transcription offers a convenient means of transcribing this abnormality, as is illustrated on the next page:

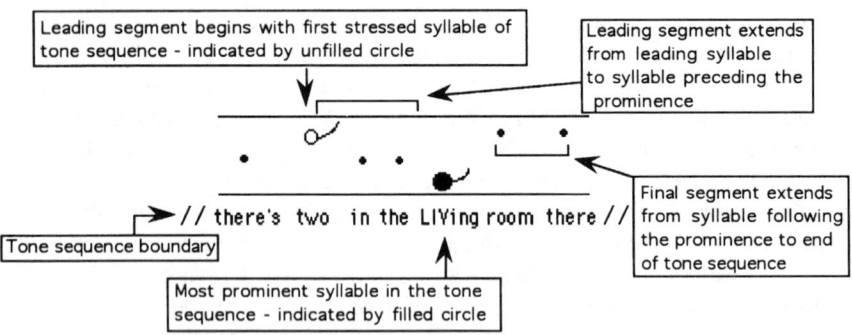

Figure 7–1. The tone sequence.

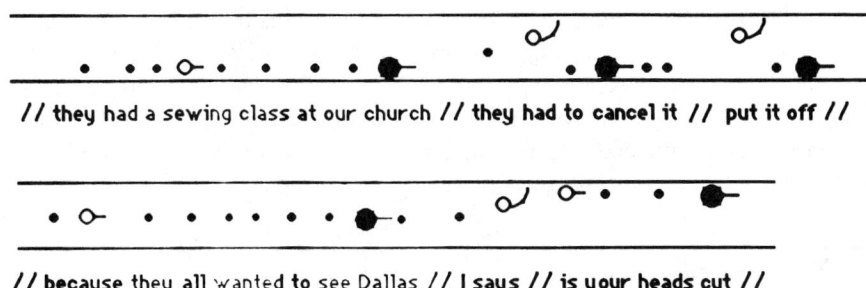

// they had a sewing class at our church // they had to cancel it // put it off //

// because they all wanted to see Dallas // I says // is your heads cut //

If the same stretch of speech were transcribed solely employing the IPA provisions for representing tones, much crucial information would be lost. The transcription would look as follows, retaining the double slash marks to indicate tone sequence boundaries:

// ↓they ↓had ↓a ↓sewing ↓class ↓at ↓our ↓church// ↑they ↑had ↓to ↓cancel ↓it// ↑put ↓it ↓off// ↑because ↑they ↑all ↑wanted ↑to ↑see ↓Dallas// ↓I↑says// ↑is ↑your ↑heads ↑cut

In particular, an IPA transcription of tones does not reflect the distribution of stresses and unstressed syllables in an utterance. In the second example above, one has no way of knowing which syllables are stressed or which are particularly prominent, for example. An interlinear transcription, however, allows degrees of stress to be recorded. The model described above permits three levels of stress to be indicated in transcription, zero stress, what we shall call "prominent stress" and "non-prominent stress." The term "prominent stress" refers to the syllables in the utterance that are perceived as being the most prominent (irrespective of the phonetic features that contribute to the prominence), and "non-prominent stress" refers to syllables which are stressed, but not particularly prominent. The graphic conventions are: an unfilled circle to represent the first stressed syllable in the sequence, a filled circle to represent the prominence, and small and larger dots to indicate unstressed and non-prominent stressed syllables, respectively. The leading syllable and prominence are joined to straight or curved lines, which indicate whether the tone is level or moving, as in examples above.

Interlinear transcription also permits the inclusion of pitch information in transcription. It is crucial to indicate the relative pitch height at which intonational components are realized, as there is evidence to suggest that inappropriate pitch of intonational components is responsible for unnatural-sounding speech

(Rahilly, 1991). We recommend a system of pitch levels transcription in which five pitch levels capture the significant areas within speakers' vocal ranges. Levels 1 and 2 are extra-low and low, respectively; level 3 is mid; level 4 is high; and level 5 is extra high. Pitch levels are assigned to the leading segment in the tone-sequence, the prominence, and the final syllable in the sequence and the levels are entered in the interlinear transcription as illustrated in:

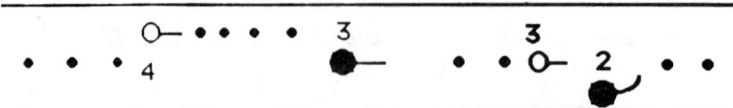

//she put a notice up on the BOARD// and we all LOOKed at it//(C10)

The information concerning the pitch height of intonational components can be used to correlate intonational structuring with aspects such as conversational structure, and cohesion, for example. Although this system of interlinear transcription has been successfully applied to the transcription of postlingually deaf speech, we imagine that it will be equally suitable for analyzing intonation in a wider range of patients.

Intensity and Speech Rate

When assessing disordered speech, the clinician will often need to indicate marked variation in the loudness and speed of speech. Although it is, of course, possible to provide instrumental measures of both of these features, we use impressionistic and relative terms from extIPA to indicate them in transcription.

Intensity is indicated by the subscript $_f$ for loud speech, $_{ff}$ for louder speech, subscript $_p$ for quiet speech and $_{pp}$ for quieter speech. The stretch of speech to which the intensity marks refer is enclosed within braces:

[xxx $\{f$ xxx $f\}$ xxx]   loud speech

[xxx $\{p$ xxx $p\}$ xxx]   quiet speech.

A similar, quasimusical, system is adopted to indicate variation in speech rate. Here, the terms are $_{allegro}$ and $_{lento}$ (both in subscript form):

[xxx $\{_{allegro}$ xxx $_{allegro}\}$ xxx] fast speech

[xxx $\{_{lento}$ xxx $_{lento}\}$ xxx] slow speech.

If we wish to record finer distinctions in speech rate, we could extend the musical analogy and use other terms such as *crescendo* or *rallentando* for example, to indicate speech that gets progressively louder or progressively slower (see W. Wells, 1992).

Conclusion

This chapter has argued that clinicians must undertake suprasegmental transcriptions if they wish to uncover the full range of abnormalities that may occur in disordered speech. It has also offered guidance for the transcription of a range of suprasegmental phenomena. Clearly, it is desirable to have recognized standards for suprasegmental transcription, along the lines of those that exist for segmental transcription. The extIPA conventions that we have explained in this chapter, along with our suggestions for emendations and additions to the IPA, represent a major step forward in establishing such standards.

CHAPTER

# of Conversation

Spoken Discourse

We turn now from the transcription of individual sounds and the transcription of words, phrases, and utterances with their prosodic features, to the transcription of larger portions of language: the text of spoken discourse. By far the most frequent kind of spoken discourse is informal conversation and whereas we shall concentrate on the most significant features of this "genre" in this chapter, we must also acknowledge the existence of other forms of spoken discourse, such as speech making, for example.

Spoken discourse may occur with only one participant, i.e. a monologue, as in a speech, or announcement; or it may involve two or many more participants, i.e. a dialogue or a more open discussion. Spoken discourse will also vary in degrees of formality; for instance, in the conduct of a wedding service, a very formal style would be expected, but when the best man gives his speech at the reception, he is expected to be very informal. Spoken discourse varies also according to the degree of preparation before the discourse ensues; many forms are scripted, such as newscasting [reading], many announcements; other forms may not be scripted, but are in some way prepared, such as the telling of a story or a joke or a service encounter in a shop; informal conversation, on the other hand, is usually completely unrehearsed. Crystal and Davy (1969, p. 102) noted that "conversation is characterized by randomness of subject-matter, and a general lack of planning."

Generally speaking, the degree of preparation is reflected in the degree of fluency in the spoken discourse. Newscasters usually speak with great fluency, as do announcers, and clergymen. To produce a transcript of such speech is relatively easy. On the other hand, spontaneous speech is characterized by an often very noticeable lack of fluency. This is not surprising when one considers the number of different tasks that such a speaker has to simultaneously engage in. As we noted in Chapter 6, Brown et al. (1980) drew attention very neatly to this multiplicity of tasks:

> In producing spontaneous speech the speaker has to decide on a topic, select the "staging" procedures for presenting his topic . . . determine what he must introduce as new and what he can taken as given, sort out the appropriate syntactic structures, select lexical items, check that his listener is following what he is saying and agreeing with it, make it clear that he wishes to continue with or to give away his turn, quite apart from speaking. (Brown et al., 1980, p. 47)

The consequence is disfluent speech, which is very much more difficult to transcribe than prepared discourse.

Two examples illustrate the discrepancy that exists between spontaneous speech and scripted speech. Speeches made in the British Houses of Parliament are recorded in detail by a team of shorthand notetakers, typists, and editors who work for the Department of the Official Report, who publish their reports daily. (The name for this service is Hansard, because the publication of records of parliamentary debate was in the hands of the Hansard family for many generations until 1889. The process is similar to the U.S. Government Printing Office publication of the *Congressional Report*.). The Hansard reports are often described as verbatim—that every word is recorded. However, they are not truly verbatim, as a good deal of editing takes place before publication. Below is a typical extract from Hansard (Slembrouck, 1992):

> As an environmental matter, 5p off the price of a gallon of unleaded petrol is welcome, not least because the leaders of the alliance will be travelling the country during the general election in a bus using this fuel. We much appreciate that contribution to our election fund.

However, what the Member of Parliament actually said is more accurately recorded in the following transcript:

> erm a_ a_ a_ as an environmental matter . the five pence off unleaded pe_ . petrol . i_ is very welcome . er not least . not least . because the leaders of the Alliance will be in fact er . travelling the country during the general election . er in a bus driven by this fuel and we very much appreciate that contribution . to our election . fund

The characteristics of typically unfluent spontaneous speech are deliberately edited out by Hansard: the hesitations, repetitions, half pronounced words, repairs, unclear sentence boundaries, and so on. Slembrouck also informs that the editing process deliberately converts the raw spoken data into literary, formal standard written English and recasts it according to parliamentary protocol. The function of Hansard is the record of messages rather than the performance of speaking: the ideational meaning is paramount, the interpersonal, the prosodic, and paralinguistic features are largely excluded. Prepublication editing of the *Congressional Record* is allowed.

However, what becomes clear from the above discussion is that spontaneous spoken discourse, even in the highest ranks of government, is marked by unfluent speech caused by the various tasks that a speaker engages in in the very act of speaking. Hesitation, repetition, reformulation, abandonment of words and of sentence syntax ("false starts"), grammatical and phonological slips, corrections to the choice of vocabulary, rephrasing, paraphrasing, asides, pauses, and a range of both vocal effects (e.g., sighing, sneering, laughing, etc.) and gestures (e.g., nodding, staring, wagging the finger) all belong to the actual performance of speaking. An accurate transcript incorporates all these features.

Hansard also arranges the contributions that members make to a debate in a neat and orderly sequence of turns and smooths over the interruptions and the simultaneous or overlapping talk that normally takes place in multisided talk. An accurate transcript also incorporates all these "untidy" features of spoken dialogue.

Another example of the discrepancy between "ideal" and real speech is the practice dialogue found in foreign language teaching coursebooks. Compare the following dialogue that has been devised to help learners practice making a transaction at a bank, with the recording of an actual transaction of a similar nature.

Following is a role play based on a cash transaction from a credit card and the conversion of the amount into U.S. dollars. The credit card customer is identified as SG and the bank cashier as GG.

SG: Good morning. I'd like to make a cash withdrawal from my credit card.

GG: Fine. I'm sorry we don't take American Express here, only Visa or Mastercard.

SG: Oh, OK. I have Visa; here you are.

GG: How much would you like?

SG: Thousand dollars please.

GG: I'm sorry, you can only make a withdrawal in pounds sterling on your credit card; we can then convert the sterling into dollars for a small commission.

SG: OK. How much is a thousand dollars in sterling?

GG: Six hundred and forty-five pounds and five pounds commission: six hundred and fifty pounds in all.

> **SG:** OK, I'll take seven hundred pounds on my Visa and convert a thousand dollars from it. What is the rate?
>
> **GG:** It's one point five five dollars to the pound.
>
> **SG:** OK.
>
> **GG:** I'll have to make a phone call to Visa.
>
> **GG:** Yes that's fine. How would you like the money?
>
> **SG:** In 20-dollar bills.

The dialog suggests that each participant waits for the other to finish before they take up their own turn, that each participant knows precisely what they will say, that both participants will keep strictly to the matter in hand, and that there are no interruptions or distractions.

Now here is a recording of an actual transaction at a bank in a similar situation. The credit card customer is identified as RP and the bank cashier as AM.

> **RP:** erm . take a θ . that amount and I wonder if you could convert it into . dollars
>
> **AM:** that amount into dollars
>
> **RP:** yeah
>
> **AM:** I'll check the rates first
>
> **RP:** OK . great . thanks
>
> **AM:** The rate this . time today is one point five two
>
> **RP:**   yeah
>
> **RP:** OK right
>
> **AM:** (inaudible) sterling before charge . will be that
>
> **RP:** So that's what is it six hundred and fifty (seven)
>
> **AM:**   six five seven . eighty nine
>
> **RP:**   OK . yeah
>
> **AM:** and the percentage - - and the percentage (unclear)
>
> **RP:** OK don't . don't worry
>
> **AM:** is one point five per cent
>
> **RP:** OK that's to be paid yeah
>
> **AM:** say that's it OK
>
> **RP:** OK fine
>
> **AM:** so it'll be six hundred and sixty seven . forty six
>
> **RP:** OK fine

AH: in sterling

RP: yeah yeah

AM: So I'll do that I'll have to ring . through to Access

RP: OK

AM: just to make sure obviously there's funds on the account

RP: that's fine yeah . OK

AM: OK

RP: that's fine

AM: (inaudible; rising tone)

RP: fine

AM: that's what I'll have to do

RP: alright that's lovely thanks very much (unclear)

AM: no problem at all
you don't want that do you.

What is immediately apparent in this transaction is the "untidiness" of the discourse, like the "untidiness" of the member of parliament's speech, compared to the "ideal" prepared dialogue. There are hesitations, false starts, repetitions, and cases of unclear syntax; but in addition, the discourse is disrupted by interventions and overlapping speech. The very cooperation between the participants disrupts the fluency of the discourse.

The last utterance of the cashier (AM) illustrates two other features of spontaneous spoken discourse. Firstly, other topics typically get included; if, in a bank transaction, as in the example, there is an interval of time while some activity is taking place, like waiting for a telephone call to be connected, the participants are quite likely to engage in small talk, perhaps about the weather, a topical news item, or an item in the immediate situation. In this particular dialogue, the cashier apparently draws attention to an object on the counter separating the pair, but it has nothing to do with the matter in hand—making a telephone call. This is an example of what Crystal and Davy (1975) called "randomness of subject matter," previously referred to. Although others, for example, Cheepen and Monaghan (1990), have questioned the appropriateness of the term "randomness"—after all, there are usually reasons for added speech that are embedded in the discourse and in the situation—spontaneous speech is characterized by these often sudden switches in subject matter.

Secondly, spontaneous spoken discourse is marked by inexplicitiness. We do not know what the *that* refers to; the referent is inexplicit. Neither do we know what *that amount* is in the opening utterance. Participants in such dialogues rely very much on the actual details in the situation—the details of the physical setting, the rapport that develops between them, the expectations of what the other knows and does, and the assumptions inherent in the particular discourse. So, for instance, one participant does not feel obliged to wait until the other has finished before initiating their own turn. Neither do the participants feel obliged to complete sentences or repair clumsy or faulty syntax or inexact vocabulary, if they feel that the message has been understood well enough; Slembrouck (1992, p. 106) noted this in parliamentary speech, too. The participants' cooperation often produces simultaneous or overlapping speech, which often hinders exact comprehension of what the other said, but often there are enough clues for them to manage without explicit repetitions. Thus, when you read such transcripts, you should not be surprized at such "loose ends"; participants do not feel obliged to explicitly tie them up.

The Reasons for Transcripts

The advent of magnetic recording tape and then its widespread availability beginning in the 1950s provided linguists with the opportunity of recording spoken discourse at length. Not only did such recordings hold the advantage of capturing long texts, but also, by careful preparation, it captured real data, not just imagined or intuited "data." Linguists were then able, for the first time in history, to investigate extended, authentic, spoken discourse and break away from the limitations of observations on brief utterances and of memory.

In the United Kingdom, in 1959, the *Survey of English Usage* was launched. Its ambitious goal was to describe the grammatical repertoire of adult educated native speakers of British English on the basis of a huge corpus that included recorded spoken discourse, with various degrees of formality. This involved the enormous task of transcribing the corpus of spoken material in a manner in which the researchers sought to incorporate every aspect of the spoken data. A prosodic transcription was evolved that sought to do justice to a wide range of prosodic and paralinguistic features (see Crystal & Quirk, 1964; Crystal, 1969).

In 1975, the Survey of Spoken English was established at Lund, Sweden with the aim of making the spoken English material of the Survey of English Usage available in print and machine-readable form. Thirty-four specimens of transcribed conversations, each lasting at least 1,200 intonation units, were printed in Svartvik and Quirk (1980). But, to reduce the complexity of the data some of the original prosodic information and virtually all of the paralinguistic information were omitted. Examples of the original detailed transcript appear in Crystal and Davy (1969).

Notice the difference in the amount of detail given in the following excerpt as presented in Figure 8–1 (Crystal & Davy, 1969, p. 97) and Figure 8–2 (Svartvik & Quirk 1980, p. 83).

1

'alleg'	A ' you got a |ₕCÓLD| ' –
'lax'	B |"NÒ| · 'just a |bit' ↑ₙSNÌFFY| cos I'm –
'dimɪn'	I |"ÀM CÓLD| and I'll ' |be all 'right 'once
'alleg piano'	I've 'warmed ÙP| – 'do I |LÒOK as
	'though I've 'got a ↑CÓLD| '
	A no I |ₕthought you SÒUNDED as 'if you
	were
'pianiss'	B ' |M̀| ' – –
'piano'	A ' |pull your CHÀIR up 'close if you WÁNT| '
	|is 'it – *(obscured speech)*
'piano'	B *' |YÈS| ' · |I'll be all 'right in a
	ₙMÍNUTE|* it's ⌊just that I'm ·

Figure 8–1. Transcript from Crystal and Davy (1969).

⁵ ‖[m̀]∎ – – – ⁶ you got a ‖CÓLD∎

⁷ – "‖NÒ∎ · ⁸ just a ‖bit △SNÌFFY∎ ⁹ cos I'm – I "‖ÀM CÓLD∎ ¹⁰ and I'll ‖be
all right 'once I've warmed ÙP∎ – ¹¹ do I ‖LÒOK as though I've got a ₐCÓLD∎
¹² no I ‖thought you SÒUNDED as if you were
¹³ ‖[m̀]∎ – – – ¹⁴ «I ‖always DÒ a bit actually∎» ¹⁵ ‖CHRÒNICALLY∎
¹⁶ – – – ‖there you ÁRE∎
¹⁷ – – – ‖ÒH∎ ¹⁸ ‖SÙPER∎
¹⁹ – – – ‖pull your CHÀIR up ▷close if you WÁNT∎ – ²⁰ ‖is it – ☆«sylls»☆
²¹ ☆‖YÈS∎ · ²² "‖I'll be all 'right in a MÍNUTE∎☆ ²³ it's ‖just that I'm
²⁴ · «‖what have you GÒT∎»

Figure 8–2. Transcript from Svartvik and Quirk (1980).

The two main aims of the *Survey of English Usage* were (a) to extend the
frontiers of linguistic description by detailed examination of the range of grammatical usage in extended discourse and of the range of prosodic and paralinguistic features in spoken discourse, and (b) to examine the characteristics of differ-

ent registers on the basis of this text-based linguistic description as a preliminary to the establishment of the study of stylistics. This text-based approach to linguistics was promoted not only by the Survey of English Usage team, which was a powerful and very influential group of British and European scholars, but also in America by the tagmemic linguists following K.L. Pike, R. Longacre and R. Grimes; D. Bolinger, too, was prominent in this respect. However, in America, the focus of linguists' attention turned away from the description of discourse following the emergence of transformational generative grammar.

Nevertheless, there emerged in America a very different new line of enquiry, which also depended on the availability of stretches of authentic speech captured on audio and later on video tapes. A group of sociologists began to investigate the nature of conversation, not from a linguistic standpoint, but from an interest in the social conventions involved in an interaction, itself. Foremost amongst these sociologists at the inception of this line of study, H. Sacks, E. Schegloff, and J.N. Schenkein should be mentioned. They and their followers, in both Britain and America, developed what came to be known as Conversation Analysis.

In Conversation Analysis, it was not linguistic description that was in focus, but the development of the interaction between the participants. Patterns of behavior were established—regular forms of organization, structures within the discourse, strategies adopted by the participants. Much attention was paid to turntaking, interruptions, and pauses. The central goal of Conversation Analysis has been stated as:

> the description and explication of the competences that ordinary speakers use and rely on in participating in intelligible, socially organized interaction. At its most basic, this objective is one of describing the procedures by which conversationalists produce their own behavior and understand and deal with the behavior of others. (Atkinson & Heritage, 1984, p. 1)

Furthermore, talk has structure from adjacency pairs—whereby one person's utterance requires a corresponding utterance from another party, as in greetings, questions, invitations—through a hierarchy of more complex and more extended transactions. Interest in individual utterances lies in the function that each performs in the whole transaction. That function can be described on two levels: at the level of speech acts—what was the person doing at that moment—thanking, apologizing, complaining, illustrating, and so on; and at the level of discourse structure—an utterance may act as an initiating or responding or follow-up move, and so on.

Transcripts of spoken discourse emanating from Conversation Analysis concentrated, understandably, not so much on linguistic detail, but on features of the behavior of the participants. They highlighted phenomena such as simultaneous and overlapping speech, latching (a following turn beginning immediately on termination of a preceding one), the timing of pauses and intervals between turns, and gaze direction. Although attention was paid to paralinguistic features, considerably less attention was paid to intonation and phonological processes like assimilation. The following scheme, as it appears in Atkinson and Heritage (1984), is basic, when you consider a comprehensive scheme such as that presented in Chapter 6.

.   A period indicates a stopping fall in tone, not necessarily the end of a sentence.

,   A comma indicates a continuing intonation, not necessarily between clauses of sentences.

?   A question mark indicates a rising inflection, not necessarily a question.

?   A combined question mark/comma indicates a rising intonation weaker than that indicated by a question mark.

!   An exclamation point indicates an animated tone, not necessarily an exclamation. (Atkinson & Heritage, 1984, p. xi)

Sometimes, normal phonological processes are highlighted as if they are in some way distinctive. R-liaison, for example, would be normal in *Justice for all*, but Potter and Wetherell (1987, p. 85) draw attention to it unnecessarily in:

Dave: What's in *Justice for=All?*

(where = means "words run together")

Similarly, weak forms of *were* and *for* would be normal in (Wetherell, 1987, p. 86)

Mark: We w're wondering if you wanted to come over Saturday, f'r dinner

where, probably, *to* could also be reduced to t', and possibly, *you* to *y'* (or *ya*).

An interest in discourse structures and speech act theory developed in Britain, too, predominantly at Birmingham (J. Sinclair, M. Coulthard, D. Brazil) and at Edinburgh (G. Brown, G. Yule). They inherited the detailed text-based description of the *Survey* team and combined it with the study of speech act theory and discourse structure. Their transcripts thus retained full prosodic information, with the intonation given in detail. An example appears in Figure 8–3.

Conventions in Transcripts

We come now to review common practices in recording features of spoken discourse in visual form. Some relevant details have already appeared in Chapter 6; the transcription of pauses, stress, length, pitch, intonation, and voice quality.

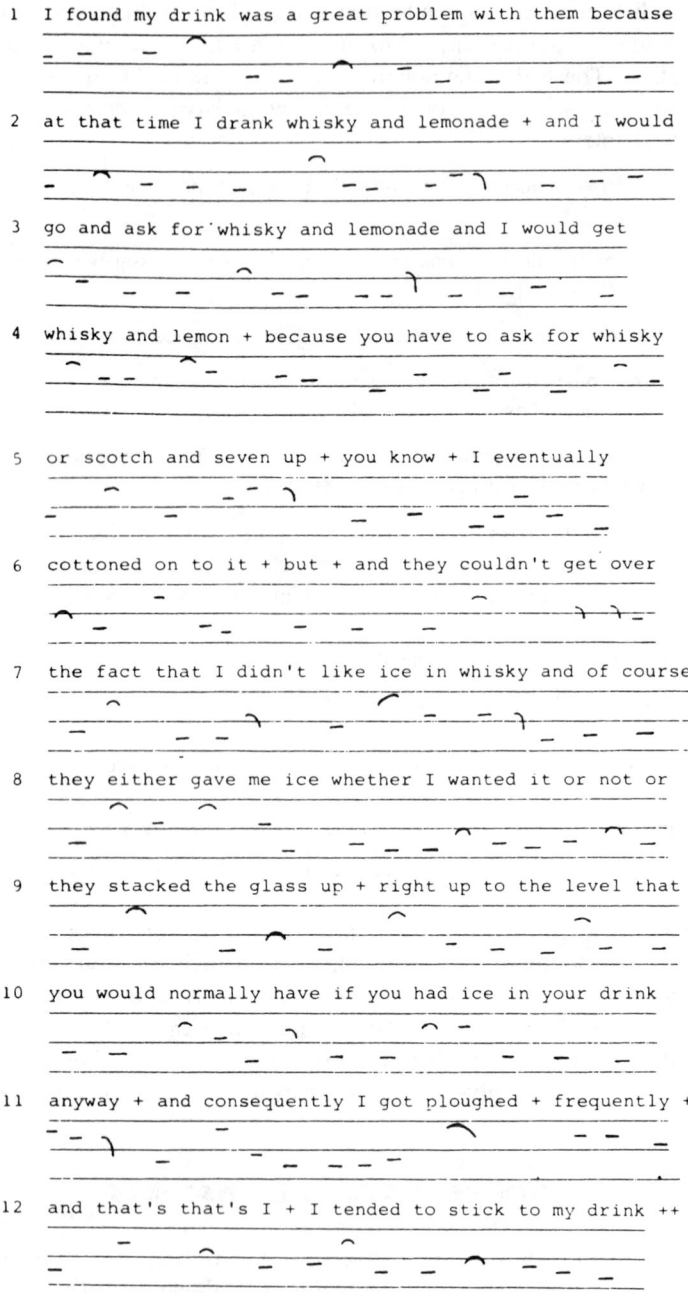

1   I found my drink was a great problem with them because

2   at that time I drank whisky and lemonade + and I would

3   go and ask for whisky and lemonade and I would get

4   whisky and lemon + because you have to ask for whisky

5   or scotch and seven up + you know + I eventually

6   cottoned on to it + but + and they couldn't get over

7   the fact that I didn't like ice in whisky and of course

8   they either gave me ice whether I wanted it or not or

9   they stacked the glass up + right up to the level that

10 you would normally have if you had ice in your drink

11 anyway + and consequently I got ploughed + frequently +

12 and that's that's I + I tended to stick to my drink ++

Figure 8-3. Transcript from Yule (1980).

The International Phonetic Association has officially approved many of these symbols and we wish to support such practice with our recommendation. But we acknowledge that there are two other major traditions: that of the (largely British) *Survey of English Usage*, and that of the (largely American) Conversation Analysis.

We also need to acknowledge that the IPA has no conventions at all covering the behaviors of participants in conversations.

We first compare the practices of the two major traditions. The two traditions can safely be represented by Crystal and Davy (Crystal & Davy, 1969, 1975) and Jefferson (1988, also Atkinson & Heritage, 1984, pp. ix–xvi).

Traditional Orthography

It is usual to present transcripts of conversation in ordinary spelling rather than phonetic or phonemic transcription. The reason for this has been the convention that what is in focus is not the pronunciation of words but rather the prosodic and paralinguistic markers of the discourse.

This has certainly been the case in the study of stylistics: It is not normally the accent or the details of segmental production that give clues to a particular genre of spoken discourse, but the presence or absence of supra-segmental characteristics, relative proportions and types. (See Tench 1988, 1990, Chapter 7, on the stylistic potential of supra-segmental features.) The preference for traditional orthography was admitted by Crystal and Davy (1969, p. 24), themselves. It was because the segmentals were less relevant for their purpose, but an understanding of the content of the discourse was essential, that they preferred a written record that was relatively easy to read. "We have tried to minimize difficulty in this matter by printing the extracts in ordinary spelling and not in phonetic or phonemic transcription in order to make them more immediately easy to read" (Crystal & Davy, 1975, p. 14).

Traditional orthography has also been preferred in the Conversation Analysis tradition. The objectives of the transcript record have been defined as "an attempt to get as much as possible of the actual sound and sequential positioning of talk onto the page, while at the same time making this material accessible to readers unfamiliar with systems further removed from standard orthography" (Atkinson & Heritage, 1984, p. 12). The system that is already somewhat "removed from standard orthography" is the system that Atkinson and Heritage attribute to Gail Jefferson mentioned above: traditional orthography modified to capture vowel qualities of colloquial (American) speech (such as *yih* for *your*, *thuh* for *the*) and elisions (such as *y'know* and *by th'way*), and accompanied by symbols and notes for the participants' behavior, pausing, paralanguage, and incidental effects (e.g., coughing, drawing breath, applause).

Two major features of conversation are ignored, however, by avoiding phonetic or phonemic transcription. One is the participants' choice of accent. Switching to, or imitating, the accent of another regional, social, or generational variety is common enough in informal conversation to justify its recognition in a written record; certainly, the choice of an alternative accent in the middle of spoken discourse is significant for the genre categorization of that discourse and for examining a speaker's intention. Such a switch can be accommodated in traditional orthography by a note, such as *(imitating Texan cowboy)* or *(working class London),* or occasional phonetic or phonemic transcription such as /gə'dai/ (representing an Australian greeting).

The second feature that is ignored in traditional orthography is the simplification system of colloquial speech: assimilation, elision, epenthesis, and liaison. These forms of simplification generally mark colloquial speech from formal and thus have stylistic significance. To a certain extent, they can be accommodated in traditional orthography, either by a note *(colloquial)* or by modifying the orthography. Elisions, of course, can be indicated by leaving a letter out, as in *marvlous* or by adapting spelling, such as *gonna*; the use of apostrophes, however, will lead to confusion with word stress (see following). If, on the other hand, a vowel that would normally be expected to be elided is nevertheless retained, it can be marked by a breve: *marvĕlous, diffĕrent, famĭly*. Epenthesis and liaison can be indicated by inserting a letter, such as *lengkth, the yanswer*. Even some assimilations have conventional spellings, *gotcha* for *got you*. However, more satisfactory would be the (if only) occasional use of phonetic/phonemic symbols, as in:

> ten green bottles
>
> [ŋ]   [m]

A comment on the presentation of weak forms is necessary at this point. In the (British) stylistics tradition, weak forms of potentially reducible words are always assumed, unless otherwise indicated, which would be by a symbol for a stressed, or a tonic syllable. Consider the following:

A: Well I 'went to 'Cardiff 'station in the /<u>mor</u>ning
to 'catch a 'train at 'half past \<u>eight</u>
'all 'rather a /<u>plea</u>sant time

B: 'on your \<u>lone</u>some

A: 'on my /<u>lone</u>some

/<u>yes</u>

'What s \<u>that</u> mean

C: 'that s \Lancashire
   for on my \tod (*laughs*)

A: \oh

(adapted from Tench, 1990, p. 689)

In line 1, *to* and *the* occurred in their weak forms /tə/ and /ðə/; this is clear by the fact that they are not stressed. In line 2, *to, a* and *at* are all unstressed and so is *past*; the latter having a weak form /pəst/ for telling the time. In lines 4 and 5, the preposition *on* is uncharacteristically stressed and that is indicated by the stress symbol. In lines 7 and 8 *is* is reduced to /s/; the apostrophe is not used, to avoid confusion with the stress symbol. In line 9, *for* is unstressed; its form here is thus /fə/ with linking /r/—it might even be reduced to /fr/; but in either case, it is left in its normal spelling, because its weak form is understood.

However, in the (American) Conversation Analysis, many of these weak forms are spelled as such. Weak *to* becomes *tuh, the* becomes *thuh, past* becomes *p'st*, and *for f'r* and so on. This kind of weak form spelling is not at all necessary if stressed syllables are consistently marked; potentially reducible forms are assumed to be reduced unless they are stressed—in which they will be marked as such.

We now review the conventions established by the two traditions for recording prosodic and paralinguistic features of spoken discourse, participants' behavior and incidental effects.

Stress

IPA and Crystal and Davy:

primary	'a
secondary	ˌa
tertiary	ₒa
none	a

Jefferson (1988) uses underlining for "emphasis" or "some form of stress, via pitch and/or amplitude." Degree of stress is indicated by the length of underlining; however, especially loud sounds are identified by capital letters:

   you couldn 'ev'n putcher hand outsI:DE the CAR

We recommend the IPA system; thus, this sample would be rendered:

   you 'couldn evn 'putcher 'hand out\side the \car

with underlining representing the tonic syllables only and accents marking the tones. The use of apostrophes for indicating the omission of a sound would be confusing; the omission of a sound can be indicated by the omission of a letter, as in *couldn*, or by a phonemic transcription, /kʊdn/. Often, elision can be "understood" as in the case of *even*.

Length

IPA uses the colon (:) to indicate distinctive degrees of length. Jefferson uses the colon to indicate length as a paralinguistic feature, too. Thus:

What ha:ppened to you

and double and triple colons for further degrees of length:

I ju::ss can't come
I'm so::: sorry re:::ally I am

Crystal and Davy refer to "drawled" syllables to indicate length as a paralinguistic feature and mark them with an equals sign above a letter:

a̿nd

Consonants that are "held" are marked by an equals sign below a letter:

b̲ut

We would recommend the IPA and Jefferson practice:

a:nd
b:ut (or bbut)

Crystal and Davy also note "clipped" syllables, that is, shorter than expected, and mark them by a dot above the vowel:

lȯt

Pauses

We have previously referred to the transcription of pausing in Chapter 6. Crystal and Davy indicate four degrees of pausing:

brief   .
unit   -
double   --
treble   ---

Duckworth et al. (1990) indicate three degrees:

short   (.)
medium length   (..)
long   (...)

Jefferson marks a short pause either by a dash or by a dot in (parentheses). But, it has been a noticeable feature of the Conversation Analysis tradition to time all but short pauses, both within an utterance and between utterances, in tenths of a second, as in:

When I was (0.6) oh nine or ten

and

Hal: Step right up
           (1.3)
Hal: I said step right up
           (0.8)
Joe: Are you talking to me.

Lehiste (1980, 1982) measured the length of pauses at "sentence" and "paragraph" boundaries and found that for one speaker the range at "sentence" boundaries stretched from 0.16 to 2.723 seconds, but the majority of them were no longer than 1.4 seconds; pauses at "paragraph" boundaries were typically at least 2.8 seconds. However, for another speaker, pauses at "sentence" boundaries averaged at 1.659 seconds, almost 20% longer than the former speaker! One is thus reminded that it is not so much actual timing that is important, but timing relative to a given speaker in a given discourse.

We recommend the Crystal and Davy scheme, as defined in Chapter 6; however we recognize that actual timing of double, treble, and longer pauses may often be worth recording and are best done in tenths of seconds enclosed in (parenthesis) as in Jefferson.

Voiced Hesitations

Again we refer first to Crystal and Davy's (1969) system of four lengths of voiced hesitation (or "audible pausing"):

brief   ə(m)
unit   əː(m)
double   əːəː
treble   əːəːəː

and then (1975) to their practice of spelling the voiced hesitations as *er, erm*, or *m*. Jefferson makes no clear reference to any conventional symbolization, but seems to "spell" voiced hesitations as *umm, uh*, and so on.

Notice the difference between American and British spellings; the British will be content with *er*, because the final *r* is not pronounced in many British accents. For that reason, it might be best to recommend the Crystal and Davy (1969) phonetic symbols.

Back Channel

Back channel is the voiced articulation that indicates a listener is paying attention to what a speaker is saying. It usually takes the form of either a bilabial nasal [m], or weakly articulated forms of *yes* (or *yeah*) and *no*, or a neutral vowel preceded by [h], as [hə], which is often doubled [həhə]. Although *yes/yeah* and *no* will no doubt be spelled, the other nonlinguistic "noises" might best be rendered as phonetic symbols.

Intonation

Again, intonation has been dealt with at some length in Chapter 6. How much of the intonation needs to be recorded will depend, as in other matters, on the purposes for which the transcript is intended. In the Conversational Analysis tradition, a bare minimum is recorded and then not consistently; the extent of the intonation system they use has been presented in the list from Atkinson and Heritage (1984).

Jefferson (1988) presented a slightly more sophisticated version:

Combinations of stress and prolongation markers indicate intonation contours. If the underscore occurs on a letter before a colon, it "punches up" the letter, i.e. indicates an "up->down" contour. If the underscore occurs on a colon after a letter, it "punches up" the colon, i.e. indicates a "down->up" contour. In the following utterance there are two pitch-shifts, the first, in "vene*e*ːr," an "up->down" shift, the second in "thouːgh", a "down->up."

J: it's only venee̱:r thou:gh,

Arrows indicate shifts into higher or lower pitch than would be indicated by just the combined stress/prolongation markers.

Punctuation markers are used to indicate intonation. The combined question mark/comma [?] indicates a stronger rise than a comma but weaker than a question mark. These markers massively occur at appropriate syntactical points, but occasionally there are such displays as:

C: Oh I'd say he's about what . five three enna ha:lf? arentchu Robert,

And occasionally, at a point where a punctuation marker would be appropriate, there is none. The absence of an "utterance-final" punctuation marker indicates some sort of "indeterminate" contour. (Jefferson, 1988, p. 194)

The system is complicated, confusing, and, in some respects, arbitrary. The development of the system has appeared rather haphazard, as if the full range of features of conversational prosody only gradually emerged in the transcribers' consciousness during a period of two decades.

The "iconic" system presented in Chapter 6 is much easier to use and read. The placement and angle of the accents is self-explanatory and there is relatively little to learn. Jefferson's examples can be converted to the following, which become much easier to read:

J: its only ve\neer /though

C: Oh Id saya hes about \what
   five three enna /half
   /arentchu Robert

The minimum that needs to be recorded are tones and accented syllables. Intonation unit boundaries can be indicated where they occur in a single line of print or can be "understood" by setting out each unit as a separate line as above. Key can be indicated by symbols or labels:

   (high)   ⌈
   (low)   ⌊
   unmarked (mid)

Other intonation components can be symbolized as in Chapter 6.

Sometimes, a noticeable change of pitch takes place within an intonation unit. A step up in pitch is marked by an upward pointing arrow and a step down by a downward pointing arrow. However, such changes of pitch must not be confused with tones on tonic syllables; thus the following transcript is confusing (Atkinson &Heritage, 1984, p. xii)

Thatcher: I am however (0.2) very ↓ fortunate

(0.4) in having (0.6) a ↑mar:vlous dep ↓uty

The first downward arrow is perhaps a low falling tone, whereas the second simply indicates the low pitch of a fall that occurred on the preceding (tonic) syllable. Thus, the text might be better interpreted as:

Thatcher: I am however . very \fortunate
- in having - a ↑ma:rvlous \deputy

Paralinguistic Features

Length, as a paralinguistic feature, has already been mentioned. Other paralinguistic features might best be labeled. Jefferson has invented some symbols for a few features: capitals for loudness, ° for quiet speech, *gh* for "gutteralness", < for hurried start, > < for speeding up and a florin sign for suppressed laughter. Other features are labeled: *cough, sniff, snorts, in falsetto, whispered.*

The range of paralinguistic features and vocal effects is too broad for a comprehensive system of symbols that are easy on the memory. An extensive list is available in Crystal and Davy (1969, p. 39) and is presented below in adapted form:

Pitch-range: *narrow, wide, monot(one), high, low, ascend(ing), descend(ing)*

Loudness: *forte, fortiss(imo), piano, pianiss(imo), cresc(endo), dimin(uendo)*

Speed: *alleg(ro), allegriss(imo), lento, lentiss(imo), accel(erando), rall(entando)*

Rhythmicality: *rhythmic, arhythmic, spiky* or *gliss(ando)* or, *stac(cato), leg(ato)*

Tension: *tense, lax, precise, slurred*

Vocal effects: *whisper, breathy, husky, creak, fals(etto), reson(ant), spread, laugh, giggle, trem(ulousness), sob, cry*

The labels are in (parentheses) and appear ahead of the stretch of discourse they relate to:

Ron: (in falsetto) I can do it now

Max: (whispered) He ll never do it

Alternatively, if the feature refers to a part of an utterance, the label appears in the margin and the relevant part of the utterance is indicated by a pair of asterisks:

```
- and I 'got my /coat    (piano)
and I got it *'all* /ready for when        (*lento)
and when he 'comes -in
'two /seats
*`smashing* you know       (*lento)
```

(adapted from Tench, 1990, p.491)

In this case, the whole of the first intonation unit is spoken softly; however, the change of speed to lento in two cases only affects certain words in the following units.

The labels for vocal effects must be positioned appropriately within the text:

Tom: I used to (*cough*) smoke a lot

Rob: (*sniff*) he thinks he s tough

Ann: (*snorts*) (Adapted from Atkinson & Heritage, 1984, p. xiii)

Unclear Speech

At times, even with the best will in the world, the task of the transcriber is made impossible, or difficult because of unclear speech. For instance, an audio recording will pick up an interference from background sound that renders a stretch of speech inaudible or incomprehensible. Also, when more than one participant is speaking, the microphone might pick up certain voices better than others. In such cases, the convention is to label a stretch of speech as (*inaudible*) or (*incomprehensible*); if it is possible to gauge the number of syllables uttered, that is likewise noted as (*5 or 6 syllables*).

If, on the other hand, the "damage" is not so serious, the transcriber may well feel that he or she can guess the wording of a stretch of unclear speech, that wording is placed in double (parentheses). The double brackets simply represent uncertainty on the part of the transcriber. If the transcriber is unable to distinguish between alternatives, both are given:

```
he 'said we 'didnt have ((enough 'air)) in the 'bedroom
                    ((an 'affair))
```

Contextual Comments

Contextual comments refer to nonlinguistic activity, which the transcriber notes as being relevant to the interpretation of the discourse. Certain kinds of activity are recorded in audiotaping, which are labeled as such in single (parentheses), as in (*telephone rings*), (*door closes*), (*sneezes*), and so on.

Jefferson has special symbols for suppressed laughter, applause and gaze direction, but these are probably best labeled in the same way as other contextual comments.

Jefferson has also special symbols for when breath is noticeably drawn in or expelled. But, again, these are probably best labeled as such when they do not interfere with articulation, as in (*sharp intake of breath*), (*slow but heavy breathing out*), and so on. If the breath stream does interfere with articulation, the phonemic details can be given immediately below the orthographic version:

> **Pam:** an ʹthis is for ʹyou (*outbreath*)
> [ɪ ɹ̥]
>
> **Dan:** (*inbreath*) ʹO ʹthank you ʹreally
> [oʊʊ̥] [ææ̥] [ɪəə̥]

(adapted from Atkinson & Heritage, 1984, p. xii)

Participants' Turn Taking

Although there is a good deal of orderliness in taking turns, participants do often produce speech that interrupts, overlaps, begins simultaneously, or latches swiftly on to the termination of the previous turn.

In orderly turn taking, the identification of each participant appears in the left margin, in turn, as in dramatic text.

Interruptions that do not substantially affect the other participant's turn are enclosed in (parentheses) in the line of print, unless they actually overlap:

> **A:** ʹWhat I ʹwant (B:but) to/*do* is ʹmake one my ˋ*self*

Overlapping speech is marked by a left-hand square bracket that ties two (or more) turns together; a right-hand square bracket marks the end of the overlap:

> **Tom:** I ʹused to ʹsmoke ⌈a \lot
> **Bob:** ⌊he ʹthinks he s ʹreal \tough
>
> **Tom:** I ʹused to ʹsmoke ⌈a \lot more⌉ than this
> **Bob:** ⌊I ʹsee ⌋

(adapted from Atkinson & Heritage, 1984, p. ix).

Other examples with interruptions and back channel follow:

A: 'What I 'want to $\lceil$ /<u>do</u> $\rceil$is 'make one my\<u>self</u>
B: $\lfloor$ but $\rfloor$

A: 'What I 'want to \<u>do</u> is 'make one my $\lceil$ \<u>self</u> $\rceil$
B: $\lfloor$ ^m $\rfloor$

The speech of two (or more) participants that begins simultaneously is marked in a similar way:

Tom: $\lceil$ I 'used to 'smoke a \<u>lot</u> when I was young
Bob: $\lfloor$ I 'used to 'smoke \<u>Camels</u>

When one participant's turn latches on quickly to the termination of another's turn, with no interval between, such "contiguous" utterances are marked by a pair of equals signs. (The following examples are all adapted from Atkinson & Heritage, 1984, p. x).

Tom: I 'used to 'smoke a \<u>lot</u>=
Bob: =he 'thinks he s 'real \<u>tough</u>

The equals signs are also used to link parts of a participant's turn when an overlap might otherwise suggest a break:

Tom: I 'used to 'smoke $\lceil$ a \<u>lot</u> more than this=
Bob: $\lfloor$ you 'used to 'smoke
Tom: =but I never in\<u>haled</u> the smoke

If more than one participant latches directly on to the termination of another's turn, this is marked by a combination of equals signs and a left-hand square bracket:

Tom: I 'used to 'smoke a \<u>lot</u>=
Bob: $\lceil$ he 'thinks he s \<u>tough</u>
       =
Ann: $\lfloor$ so did \<u>I</u>

If a participant latches directly on to the termination of an overlapping turn, a similar combination with a right-hand square bracket is required:

Tom: I 'used to 'smoke a \lot ⎤
                                          ⎥ =
Bob: I \see ⎦

Ann: =so did \I

A Worked Example

We now apply these transcript conventions to the dialogue, given above, of the cash transaction at a bank. We present it in traditional orthography, but with phonetic symbols where relevant to indicate simplifications; there is no obvious switch in accent during the course of this dialogue. Stresses are indicated. There happens to be no instance of paralinguistically lengthened syllables. Pauses, voiced hesitation, and intonation are indicated in full. Notes on a few cases of other paralinguistic features are given, as are a few contextual comments. Back channel is transcribed. Details of the participants' turn taking are also transcribed.

The turns are numbered for ease of reference. Intonation units within each turn are presented on separate lines; this makes it easier to show the extent of paralinguistic features. RP is the customer, AM the bank cashier.

1 RP: Can you əm . take a th . 'that a/mount
             and I 'wonder if you could con'vert it into . \dollars
                                    [g]
2 AM: 'that a'mount into \dollars=
3 RP: =\yeah   (low, soft)
4 AM: I ll 'check the 'rates /first
5 RP: O\k
             \great   (low)
             \thanks
(46 secs . AM leaves)
6 AM: the 'rate 'this . 'time to/day   (high)
7 RP: yeah   (narrow)
6 AM: is 'one point 'five \two=
                [m]
8 RP: =O/k
             ⎡\right   ⎤
9 AM: ⎣(inaudible)⎦ 'sterling before /charge   (low)
             . will be /that   (low)

10 RP: so 'that s
             \<u>what</u> is it   (low, soft, allegro)
             'six 'hundred ⎡and 'fifty ((seven))⎤
11 AM: ⎣'six 'five 'seven .⎦ 'eighty /<u>nine</u>
12 RP: o\<u>k</u>
             .\<u>yeah</u>
13 AM: and the per\<u>cent</u>age
(14 secs)

             and the per˘<u>cent</u>age (inaudible; traffic noise)(low, soft)
14 RP: O\<u>k</u>
             dont . dont /<u>worry</u>   (narrow, soft)

(19 secs)
15 AM: is 'one point 'five per \<u>cent</u>
               [m]

16 RP: O\<u>k</u>
             that s to be \<u>paid</u>
             /<u>yeah</u>   (soft)

(4 secs)
17 AM: Say \<u>that</u> s it   (soft)
             O/<u>k</u>=   (soft)

18 RP: =O/<u>k</u>
             \<u>fine</u>   (low)

(14 secs)
19 AM: 'So it ll be 'six hundred and sixty 'seven . 'forty 'six
20 RP: O-<u>k</u>
  RP: /<u>fine</u>
19 AM: in /<u>ster</u>ling=
21 RP: =\<u>yeah</u>   (low, soft)
             /<u>yeah</u>   (low, soft)

(4 secs)
22 AM: So I ll 'do /<u>that</u>=
             = I ll 'have to 'ring . 'through to /<u>Access</u>

23 RP: O/<u>k</u>

24 AM: 'just to make 'sure /<u>obvi</u>ously
             there s 'funds on the ac\<u>count</u>

25 RP: thats \<u>fine</u>   (low)
             \<u>yeah</u>   (low, soft)
             O\<u>k</u>
26 AM: O/<u>k</u>

27 RP: thats \fine

28 AM: ⌈ (inaudible; rising tone) ⌉

           | |=

29 RP: ⌊ \fine   ⌋

30 AM: ='that s 'what I ll have to \do

31 RP: al/right

             'that s \lovely

             'thanks very \much

             ⌈if you (inaudible) ⌉

32 AM: ⌊ 'no 'problem at \all⌋   (low, allegro)

             . you 'dont 'want ./that do you   (high, allegro)

The recording was made by audio cassette placed on the counter in a bank with the consent of the cashier. Traffic noise fills the background and one point (turn 13) obscures the cashier's low, soft utterance. Other people's voices often intrude, too. In the following commentary, the terminology used to describe the development of the discourse is that of Francis and Hunston (1992).

After consent has been obtained to record the dialogue, RP initiates his request, abandons his first attempt at wording it, repairs it with an inexplicit *that*, and completes his intended message with a second intonation unit. The colloquial style is indicated by the assimilation of the *d* of *could*. The pause before *dollars* is difficult to explain, but is nevertheless typical of unrehearsed colloquial speech.

The cashier confirms RP's intentions and RP concurs; his turn latches directly on to the cashier's. AM then starts a new move and uses a rising tone which suggests he intends to follow up with more information; which he does not do. RP concurs (turn 5) with *Ok*, then *great* on a low key. The low-pitched *great* acts as a terminator of the move, but RP obviously wants to sound appreciative and adds *thanks* with a degree of prominence, by a return to a higher key (not labeled, but inferrable).

After 46 seconds of absence from the counter, AM signals a new topic by choosing high key (turn 6). RP's back channel does not interfere with AM's turn, which continues on a lower key (not labeled). That AM's style is colloquial is indicated by the assimilation of /n/ of *one*. As RP confirms, his speech overlaps that of AM's next utterance which is rendered inaudible. The low key of that turn indicates that that topic is soon to be concluded; however it is not allowed to run to its full conclusion—note that the second unit in turn 9 has an incomplete (rising) tone—because of RP's intervention (turn 10).

RP, in turn 10, interrupts himself with *what is that*? spoken quickly, quietly and in a low key, which is typical of the way a speaker switches communication with the addressee to a communication with themself; whereas the rest of that turn is addressed to the cashier, that one intonation unit is a case of self-consultation.

The cashier confirms RP's calculation and dominates the overlapping speech in the confidence that his calculation will carry authority. RP concurs.

The cashier then initiates a new informing move (turn 13) with a 14-second gap, presumably to operate a calculator; the repetition is on a low key and continues too quietly to be understood. RP seeks to reassure AM that he is not worried. However, AM perseveres and the sentence begun in turn 13 is eventually completed, at least 33 seconds later, in turn 15.

In turn 16, RP acknowledges AM's provision of information and moves on to an enquiry. The quietness of the speech suggests a kind of acquiescence. The next turns, after a further checking with the calculator, follow quickly and quietly, reaching low key for the termination of that move.

The cashier, after further calculations, initiates a new informing move, which is interrupted and then concluded by RP's repeated concurring, again finishing low and quiet.

There then appears to be 4 seconds for reflection. AM's turn (22) contains an offer which is swiftly followed by a statement of what he is thus obliged to do and an explanation (turn 24) of why he has to do it. Again this move is interrupted and then completed by RP's concurring, which finishes in low key, quietly.

AM seeks confirmation, despite all RP's previous concurring, with a high rising tone, presumably to emphasize his role in servicing the request. RP then appears so anxious to concur that he obliterates AM's turn (28); AM also appears anxious to confirm RP's intentions by latching turn 30 to RP's concurring *fine*.

RP follows up with a rather elaborate set of intonation units that act as confirmation, concurrence, and an attempt to express deference, which is, however, obscured by AM's conclusion of the whole transaction. The rapidity of speech in the formula *No problem at all*, in low key, signals the end of the transaction.

The utterance that follows is on a high key which signals a new topic, indeed a new transaction. The use of the negative in the enquiry and a checking tag indicate that AM expects the response to be negative. There is, in fact, no response, and so the second transaction is completed in a single turn. The speed of articulation in the turn is an indication also that the speaker expected that the new transaction would not extend for long.

Transcripts of Aphasic Subjects' Conversations

The conventions for transcribing the conversation of people with disordered speech, such as aphasic subjects, is basically no different from those for normal conversations. The transcripts simply become the records of the disordered conversation itself. Conversation may become disordered in three areas: cohesion or lack of it within a stretch of discourse; the maintaining, or flouting, of the principle of cooperation amongst the participants, and the skills or lack of them in executing the strategies involved in developing a conversation.

Cohesion has been defined as the set of linguistic resources that every language has for linking one part of a text with another to produce discourse (see Halliday, 1994, p. 309). They are the means by which users of the language show the integrity of a discourse. "Cohesion occurs when the interpretation of some element in the discourse is dependent on that of another" (E.M. Armstrong, 1991, p. 41). The linguistic resources for cohesion in conversation are lexical, grammatical and intonational.

Lexical cohesion is the deployment of lexical items in a discourse. Lexical items may be deployed, for instance, to maintain reference to the identity of an item in the discourse, either by repetition of words—for instance, *amount* and *dollars* are both repeated in utterance 2 in the dialogue above—or by using a synonym, a superordinate, or a general word. Lexical items also display collocation, that is, the conventional association of words—for instance, *sterling* collocates with *dollars*, *rates* with *percentages*, *funds* with *account*, and so on.

Grammatical cohesion is the grammatical means by which a discourse is made to hang together. The use of pronouns, for instance, within and across utterances, ties them together; *it* in line 2 ties that utterance to the previous one. Both participants used demonstratives heavily to achieve cohesion. Definite articles perform the same kind of function. (Lessor & Milroy (1993, p. 6) report on the particular difficulties that deixis and definiteness present to aphasics.) Ellipsis—the omission of part of a grammatical structure—displays cohesion too, as the interpretation of what is uttered depends crucially on recognizing the context.

Intonation also provides evidence of the integrity of a discourse, primarily through the structure of new and given information (Halliday, 1994, pp. 298–299; Tench, 1990, pp. 185-188):

A: d'you 'take /<u>sugar</u>
B: I 'gave \<u>up</u> 'sugar
  a little \<u>while</u> ago

The fact that *sugar* does not take the most prominent syllable in the first part of B's reply shows that it is being treated as given information—which, itself, means that the reply can only make sense in a specific context.

E.M. Armstrong (1991) is an introduction to the study of cohesion in aphasic discourse. She first presents a sample of normal speech obtained by using a cartoon strip designed to elicit a narrative, and then compares two samples of aphasic speech with it. The sample of normal speech was presented as:

Text A

1. A *little girl's kitten* was *caught* in a *tree*
2. The *child was* very *upset*
3. Because *she* couldn't *get it down*
4. *A man came along*
5. And *tried* to *get* the *cat down*
6. *He climbed* the *tree*
7. But before *he reached* the *cat*
8. *It jumped down*
9. And the *child was happy*
10. *He* then *crawled back* along the *branch*
11. But got *caught himself* on a *twig*
12. And the *fire brigade* had to *come*
13. And *get* the *man down*

The italics represent lexical and grammatical items that display cohesion. (Intonational cohesion was not discussed by Armstrong.)

Now follows the attempt by one aphasic patient to narrate the same story. The story is still easily recognizable as the same, but it is less easy to follow. This is not only because of the lack of grammatical and lexical items, but the cohesion is not as effective. The use of the word *business*, for instance, seems to be a poor choice as a general word; notice also that no synonyms are used.

Text B

1. There *was kitten up* in the *tree*
2. And the *little girl tried* to . . .
3. *wanted it down*
4. And a *chap came along*
5. And *he . . . he tried* to *get it down*
6. *He* didn't *work too good*
7. Because *he upset* the *business*
8. And the *kitten jumped down*
9. And *left him hanging up* in the *tree there before*
10. But *he* should have *had* a *guard*
11. *Somebody come* to have *done it*
12. Should have *somebody else . . . proper one*

The third text is that of another aphasic, who is clearly less able to achieve cohesion other than by repetition and pronouns.

Text C

1. Well *he goes*
2. *It goes off* with a *chap* and *his sister*
3. And *he sees* a *cat on top of* the *hen* . . . no
4. *He sees* a *cat on top* of the (what do you call it) . . . *tree*
5. And *she's down there*
6. And *she gets down there*
7. And *she* and the *chap comes up*
8. And *she* and *he gets* to the *tree*
9. And then *he's there*
10. And *he throws* the *cat down* to *her*
11. And then the *little girl* . . . and the *fireman are there getting*

The transcripts follow the same conventions as transcripts of normal speech (although in these cases, much simplified and clearly edited). They are merely the means for recording cohesion difficulties and disorders.

A second area of disorder in the conversation of aphasics is compliance with the maxims of conversational cooperation (Grice, 1975). The four maxims for effective collaboration in the construction of conversation relate to quantity (i.e. , giving the right amount of information—not too much, not too little), quality (i.e., giving the right account the information or truthfulness), manner (i.e., giving information with clarity and orderliness) and relevance.

In the following text, the maxims of quantity and relevance appear to be flouted:

1. **T.** is it raining today
2. **P.** er (cough) it's quite (cough) pardon / no it never put me off (uhuh) no I was quite happy (right) even if it was raining and then I'd see it would cloud away and would be blue (OK) and you're happy (yes) all over again I always used to feel good about things
3. **T.** OK and the last one /is it Monday today
4. **P.** Monday/ that's the beginning (right) it is *the* beginning
5. **T.** is it Monday today
6. **P.** it's a Monday
7. **T.** is it Monday today
8. **P.** oh this one you mean

9. T. Today

10. P. oh now this is fourth fifth February/ its about the fourth fifth is it now.... (Hawkins, 1989)

S. Edwards & Garman (1989) noted how one patient became a compulsive talker as a strategy for not yielding the floor and thus revealing comprehension problems.

It might be noted however, at this point that Lesser and Milroy (1993) have observed how people respond in institutional talk as compared to ordinary conversation. In the former, one participant takes the lead, as in an interview between a doctor and a patient, or a person seeking information of a policeman, or a teacher in school, and so on. The other person's responses are inevitably constrained by the lead taken by the dominant participant. Many of the examples of aphasics' conversation published in the literature are actually obtained in therapist-patient institutional talk. In their discussion Lesser & Milroy (1993, pp. 160–166) quote one aphasic's personal observation:

> "talking with [pi:θ] (people)/ it's alright like my, my old wife at home [θ]/ when he say to me [θ] about it and I could talk beautiful/ . . . y'know/ it's funny, init/ y'can't talk with everybody—this is , this is what it's about [θ]"

The cooperative principle in the construction of conversation takes on another dimension of meaning when an unaffected participant engages an aphasic participant in conversation. Normally in conversation, the participants help each other out, but it is inevitable that the burden of collaboration falls more heavily on an unaffected participant when conversing with an aphasic. Two examples are reproduced from Lessor & Milroy (1993, p. 180):

(i) APHASIC: I /and of course she was saying today/ well eventually/ I says no no no I says they won't/ I says

NON-APHASIC: who's this/ Deirdre was saying this today was she?

APHASIC: yes yes/ half past ten on a Friday

(ii) APHASIC: and er Joan/ she was erm/ he was a what was it/ come on

NON-APHASIC: she was an air hostess?

APHASIC: yes/ a what

NON-APHASIC: an air hostess

APHASIC: yes but in the airforce

NON-APHASIC: oh/ was she an air traffic controller

APHASIC: that's right

This leads to consideration of the third area of potential difficulty in aphasics' conversation: strategies involved in the actual production of conversation. The strategies include opening and closing, turntaking, embedding, repairs, discourse signals, and nonlinguistic activity.

The opening in our worked banking example is missing, but presumably at the opening of a transaction between a customer and a bank cashier there would be at least a greeting. At its closing, there is likely to be an expression of thanks, acknowledgment, and farewell. In the worked example, there is a temporary closing in turn 32: *no problem at all,* which is a common formulaic expression of confidence in being able to perform the promised service. It is claimed that aphasic speakers are expected to be relatively skilled in routine linguistic behavior of this kind (Lessor & Milroy, 1993, p. 204).

It is also claimed that aphasic speakers seem on the whole to handle the skills of turn taking effectively, except in the case of rapid repairs at turn beginnings (Lesser & Milroy, 1993, p. 192). An example of the latter appears below. Typically, an exchange consists of an initial utterance and a response—a sequence often referred to as an adjacency pair—with an optional follow-up. If the response is silence, it is usually interpreted as a negative, as in:

A: I was 'hoping 'you'd ne 'able to \help me

B: (2 secs)

A: Oh \'well
    I 'thought I'd ˇask

In the following extract, the therapist (T) construes the 1-second pause as a negative, whereas the patient (P) had actually chosen an inappropriate lexical item earlier (*pre-war*) but was unable to repair quickly enough to forestall P's misinterpretation.

1. **P:** (1.0) we (.) ma ma ma (2.4) married (8.0) pre-war=
2. **T:** =mhm
3. **P:** (.) we got married=
4. **T:** =yem mhm did you go away for the war
5.   (1.0)
6. **T:** no (.) you didn't=
7. **P:** =no no no (1.0) er (2.5) um (13) [4 syll] (7.0) [3 syll] married=
8. **T:** =mhm
9. **P:** (2.5) [5 syll]=
10. **T:** =mhm (Lesser & Milroy, 1993, p. 196)

A greater difficulty for aphasics in the construction of exchanges appears to be the embedding, or nesting, of one exchange within another. There appears to be a significant absence of such in aphasic speech (Lesser & Milroy, 1993, p. 199).

Repairs, in general, constitute a major difficulty, because of the need for speed and precision. The following extract is from a conversation between a student therapist (T) and an aphasic patient with severe lexical retrieval problems:

1. **T:** Did you stay in this country=
2. **P:** =no *no*
3. **T:** *you went* abroad=
4. **P:** = *no no* no we (and.1) [teriz] (2.4)
5. **T:** is it [teteri] terrors
6. **P:** (.) no (2.0) um (6.4) [4 syll] (3.1) ah (4.0)
7. **T:** are you trying to tell me the name of a country=
8. **P:** =no no=
9. **T:** =no=
10. **P:** =no I've (4.1) (Lesser & Milroy, 1993, p. 192)

This repair sequence, despite the patient's ability to participate in the turn-taking procedure, was unsuccessful. It emerges, after another 50 turns, that the patient had intended to say *Yes* at turn 4 above.

The following two extracts are conversations between pairs of aphasic sufferers at a stroke club. In the first, the word sought is *embroidery*, and in the second, *bat*, even though it has been already articulated successfully:

1. **B:** er er
2. **M:** [krou] cherries
3. **B:** [kou] yes uh (.) no
4. **M:** [kou]
5. **B:** no
6. **M:** crocheries?
7. **B:** (.) er(3.0) er oh dear [kos] er (2.0) oh dear
8. **M:** I ca:nt
9. **B:** [les] (.) [boi boidi]
10. **M:** er broi:dery
11. **B:** broidery (.) yes (.) oh dear

1. **G:** and the the one the bat in the er [pand] pant er pant
2. **R:** pant?
3. **G:** the er erm
4. **R:** (.) ball is eh (2.0) oh the tennis
5. **G:** yeh (3.0) the er (*picks up paper and draws diagram of table tennis table, bats [paddles], and balls*)

6. **R:** (.) yeh (6.0) yeh (.) cash with order (2.0)
7. **G:** what's the er?
    (3.0)
8. **R:** oh
    (2.0)
9. **G:** the small (*cups two hands together*)
10. **R:** (.) yes (*both laugh*)
    (4.0)
11. **G:** the small [baʔ bak]
12. **R:** bat (1.0) bat
13. **G:** uh bat
14. **R:** bat
15. **G:** yeah er small and uns
16. **R:** small ball (*G points to drawing*)
17. **G:** er the inch ball (.) yeah yeah
18. **R:** yes yes
    (3.0)
19. **G:** yes
    (5.0)
20. **R:** yes (*G puts pen and paper down and laughs*) (Lesser & Milroy, 1993, p. 215–216)

The second of these extracts illustrates the rather excessive use of discourse signals such as *oh, yeh/yes*, which is often characteristic of aphasics' conversations. Although these signals are relatively empty semantically, they are extremely important in the maintenance of conversation. Signals like *well, so* (see turns 19 and 22 in the worked example above), *now, then, y'know*, and of course, *no* are relatively effortless ways of maintaining a degree of participation in a dialogue.

That same extract demonstrates the importance for aphasics of non-linguistic activity to compensate for loss of linguistic production. Such activity in normal conversation often serves as a complementary mode of communication. When it does, it is entered in the transcript as contextual comments. However, it seems inevitable that a linguistically impaired participant in a conversation will rely more heavily on gestures, acting, drawing, pointing, and the like, rather like a stranger who does not know much of the language of a community in which they find themselves.

We conclude with a transcript of a conversation involving a patient (P), her husband (H) and daughter (D), and a student therapist (T)

1. **T:** and write it down
2. **P:** yes yes and er er er er er about half past (.) twelve (.) you get er
    your (*demonstrates exercises*) er er er oh dear

    (1.0)
3. **H:** exercises
4. **D:** dad
5. **P:** exe (*waves hands*) (*all laugh*) ex (*all laugh*)
6. **H:** I know what she's trying to say you see (*laughter*)
7. **P:** exercises (*demonstrates exercises*) that's like this (.) you know
    (*waves hand*) and er about five (.) after that it be dinner time (2.0)
    then we get our dinner (1.0) and then come back and then (3 syll)
    they that they play um er (7.0; *writes 'S' in the air; continues to
    make a waving gesture;* 8.0) er (4.0) er er to do with er ah er
    scribble ah scrabble scrabble
8. **S:** scrabble
9. **T:** uhuh
10. **P:** yes (Lesser & Milroy, 1993, p. 214)

Future Developments in Transcription

Throughout this book we have stressed the importance of narrow phonetic transcription when describing disordered speech. However, as we have also pointed out, narrow transcription is not only difficult, but can present problems of reliability. That is to say, different transcribers may not agree on how to transcribe specific parts of an utterance and, indeed, the same transcriber may be inconsistent between one attempt and another at transcription. Future developments in phonetic transcription—particularly within the clinical field—should aim, therefore, at minimizing these discrepancies without abandoning the goal of a narrow, detailed transcription. In this chapter, we discuss one specific development in this area.

Instrumental Description

Modern phonetic investigations have tended to move somewhat away from traditional impressionistic transcriptions towards the use of instrumental analysis of speech. A large variety of instrumental techniques are available (see, for example, Code & Ball, 1984; Ball & Code, in press), and they are suitable for the analysis of articulatory, acoustic, and auditory/perceptual aspects of phonetics. The advantages of instrumental analyses include that they tend to do away with issues of reliability, in that, as long as the same piece of apparatus with the same settings is used for a given sample, the resultant analysis should be the same regardless of who undertook it or when.

This is not to suggest that instrumental techniques are the answer to all problems of phonetic description: They do not give us "the right answer." To a lesser or greater extent, all phonetic equipment simplifies the incoming data, through, for example, filtering the acoustic data or through the number of times per second an articulatory posture can be measured. Further, some of the resultant data displays or readouts may not be easy to measure to an absolute degree of interscorer reliability, although the differences may be very small.

A further problem with instrumental phonetics is that the equipment may not always be where the speaker is, and although some equipment may be useable with tape-recorded input, not all is. For speech-language pathologists, the use of more sophisticated equipment may be beyond the level of facilities provided by their clinics, and time pressure may preclude regular, in-depth analysis of speech samples instrumentally.

Nevertheless, what we are beginning to see is a move towards the use of instrumental phonetic analysis as an aid to more traditional impressionistic transcription. Developments are taking place whereby instrumental phonetic evidence is being referred to for help in resolving disagreements in transcription (see, for example, Klee & Ingrisano, 1992). Future developments in phonetic transcription for speech-language clinicians will surely lie in this area, and we will describe in some detail one of the first systems to address this. First, we need to know a little more about some of the important pieces of phonetic instrumentation that might be used in this synthesis of instrumental and impressionistic description.

Acoustic Instrumentation

Instrumentation to investigate sound waves has been available to phoneticians since the 1940s. In recent times, such instrumentation has been integrated into personal computers and so has become quick and easy to use, as well as comparatively cheap. There are currently acoustic analysis systems available for operation with IBM-format PCs and for Apple Macintosh computers.

There are three main aspects of the acoustic wave that have been investigated through phonetic instrumentation: time, frequency, and intensity. Clearly, speech events take place in time, and in many speech disorders (such as stuttering) relative timing of one aspect of speech as opposed to others can be of great interest. However, in speech research one requires the ability to examine very small differences in timing. For example, the aspiration following the plosive burst found in many voiceless plosives in English lasts for perhaps 100 msecs and some important timing differences may be even shorter than this.

Characteristics of the complex sound waves that make up speech are measured in hertz (Hz), which are equivalents to cycles per second—that is, the number of complete repetitions of the wave in 1 second. This aspect is referred to as frequency, and the fundamental (i.e., basic) frequency of the voice at any one time is the acoustic correlate of pitch (the linguistic use of which is termed intonation). Measurements of frequency are very useful, therefore, in investigating intonation, for example, in the speech of the deaf (see Chapter 7).

However, because of the complex nature of speech sound waves, phoneticians can also measure the frequency of other aspects of speech. Vowel sounds, for example, typically display three (and more) significant bands of intense frequency (termed "formants"). Measurements of these can help in identifying vowel sounds that we may find difficult to transcribe. All sound types have typical frequency patterns (see Ball, 1993), and so an analysis of frequency helps in the description of phonetic data.

Intensity is the acoustic correlate of loudness and is the amount of acoustic energy utilized in any particular band of frequency in the sound wave. An analysis of intensity can help in comparing the relative loudness of speakers or speech sounds. It is also used in analyzing frequency, as the formants referred to show up because they are more intense areas of frequency.

The sound spectrograph has traditionally been the instrumentation used to analyze speech acoustics (see Farmer, 1984, in press). As noted above, sound spectrography is usually now found as part of a microcomputer package (as with the Kay Elemetrics CSL system). The most commonly used setup for a spectrograph involves a printout that plots time (in msecs) along the x-axis and frequency (in Hz) on the y-axis. Intensity is shown by the relative darkness of the frequency traces. A typical spectrogram is shown in Figure 9–3. Other settings are available, however. A single moment in the speech wave can be selected, and frequency plotted against intensity. Fundamental frequency measures (F_0) can often be worked out, as well as measures of pitch perturbation: jitter and shimmer.

Articulatory Instrumentation

A wide range of instrumentation is available to measure articulation. For example, airflow and degrees of orality and nasality can be measured via a variety of mask-based equipment (see Anthony & Hewlett, 1984; Zajac & Yates, in press), with vocal fold activity having been investigated through the use of the electrolaryngograph (see Abberton & Fourcin, 1984, in press). However, if one is mostly interested in place and manner of articulation, one must either use a variety of expensive imaging techniques (such as radiography, ultrasound, magnetic resonance imaging, etc.; see Ball & Gröne, in press) or some method of measuring tongue contact patterns on the roof of the mouth.

Electropalatography (EPG: see Hardcastle & Gibbon, in press) is a technique that utilizes an artificial palate fitted with a large numer of electrodes to measure tongue contact patterns in speech over time. Every time the tongue touches the roof of the mouth, the electrodes in that area fire, and as the system samples data very rapidly (normally 100 times a second), very detailed information on tongue movements can be obtained. The modern EPG systems operate in "real-time," which means the patterns are displayed instantaneously on the computer screen (see Figure 9–3 for a typical EPG display).

EPG cannot, of course, give information about consonants (such as bilabials, pharyngeals) that do not involve tongue contact between the alveolar ridge and the soft palate, nor about those sounds (such as low vowels) that involve no kind of lingual contact. Nevertheless, EPG has been found to be very useful in the investigation of articulation disorders and can also be a most effective training tool in the clinic.

As with spectrography, one can use EPG to provide normative data about articulation types, against which we can compare disordered speech data. Clearly, if one could use a database of both spectrographic and EPG information on normal and disordered speech, one would have a powerful instrumental phonetic tool to aid in transcription of atypical speech production. In the next section we discuss such a development.

The Kay Elemetrics Phonetic Tutorial Program

The current IPA Transcription Tutorial, Model 4335 program running on the Kay Computerized Speech Lab™ (CSL) has been designed to assist students of phonetics, linguistics, and speech science to learn and use the International Phonetic Alphabet. This program provides facilities for learning the IPA symbols and how to use them in transcription through exercises in annotating, describing and identifying phonetic impressions of a wave form that is graphically represented on the display screens.

The IPA font set that is installed into the program includes consonant and vowel symbols, segmental diacritics, suprasegmental symbols, and transcription boundary markers. The basis for the font set is the International Phonetic Alphabet (revised to 1989) as published in the *Journal of the International Phonetic Association* (IPA, 1989). In addition, a number of other symbols that have traditionally been used for phonetic transcription have been included in the set. All symbols are accessed for transcription by selecting them individually from a graphically represented symbol list in which the symbols are listed in order of their assigned IPA numbers as established by the IPA in 1989.

The program makes use of a subset of CSL commands and functions to enable access, display, and audio monitoring of sampled data files, with automatic display of palatograms if the files were created using the Palatometer. Spectrograms are also automatically computed and displayed and all view screens are linked together to enable coordinated data display and cursor movement.

An important feature of the IPA Transcription Tutorial program is the display of the IPA Consonant Chart and Vowel Chart, along with a list of other symbols that are not traditionally displayed in the format of a chart. Supported by speech data that may be listened to or displayed spectrographically, these charts and the "Other Symbols" list are a key aspect of the IPA Transcription Tutorials in that they may be used to introduce the student to basic pronunciations associated with the consonant and vowel symbols.

The following figures illustrate some of the screens available in the current IPA Transcription Tutorial Program. Figure 9–1 is the Consonant Chart, which, as noted, includes more symbols than the IPA 1989 revision chart. It allows users to select, for example, voiceless nasals, voiceless approximants, and dental and alveolar place of articulation.

With this chart displayed, the user may use the mouse button to compare audio samples along the place of articulation axis, selecting items in one of the vertical columns. Similarly, comparing audio samples along the manner of articulation axis is done by systematically selecting items from one of the horizontal rows. Voicing can be sampled by selecting the left hand (voiceless) or right hand (voiced) symbol of a pair.

The Vowel Chart in Figure 9–2 can be similarly used to compare audio samples of different vowel qualities, including Cardinal Vowel values, as well as the IPA "spare symbols" for lax vowels.

An important application for the program is to aid transcribers in assigning IPA symbols to their own data. This data can be analyzed by the CSL to provide a spectrographic and palatographic display. This display can then be compared with stored data in the transcription program by clicking on the relevant IPA symbol at any point during the utterance under analysis. The stored samples (that provide displays from two different phoneticians for each item) can then be viewed on the screen.

Figure 9–3 illustrates an analysis of a sample provided by a user, with the palatographic trace of a point towards the end of the utterance, as shown by the cursor, which also indicates the relevant point on the spectrographic trace and waveform. The user can then compare waveform, spectrographic trace, and palatographic trace from the stored samples by clicking on the relevant symbol to bring these up to the screen, and finding the closest match.

The final stage is for the user to enter the relevant IPA symbol into the window provided.

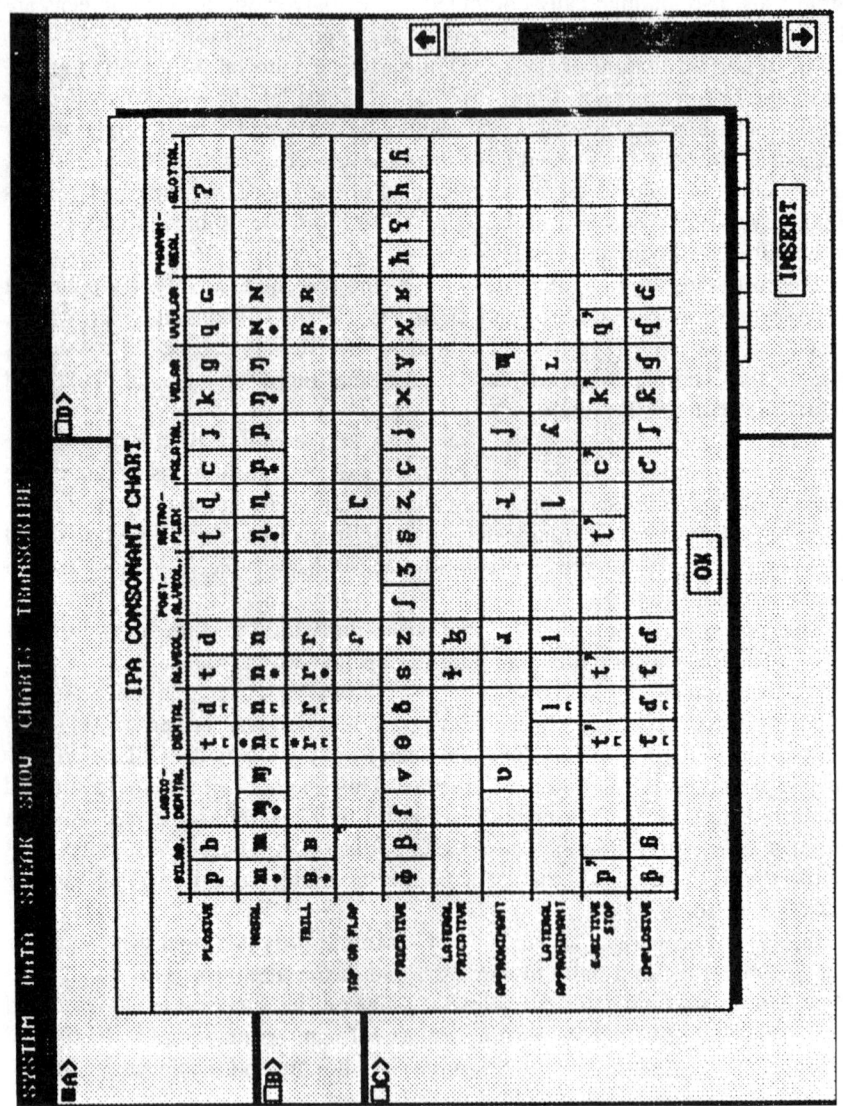

Figure 9-1. The IPA Tutorial Consonant Chart.

192

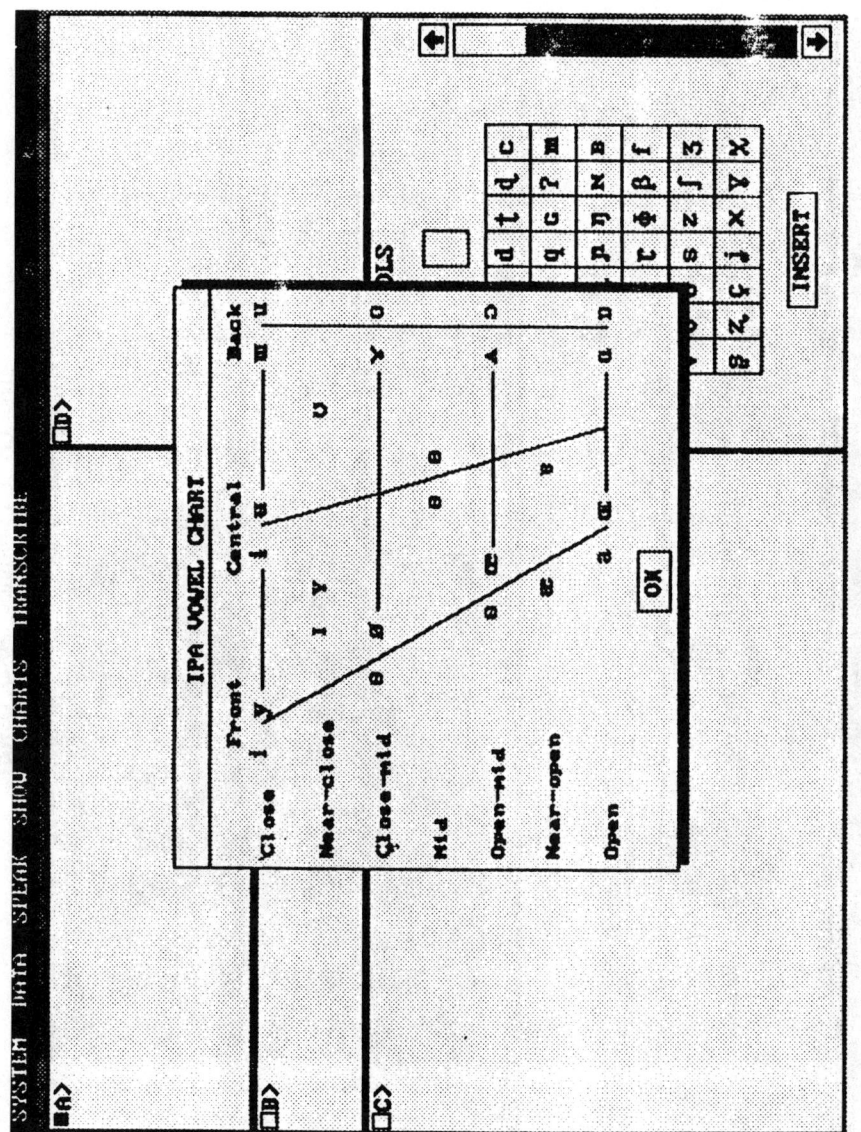

Figure 9-2. The IPA Tutorial Vowel Chart.

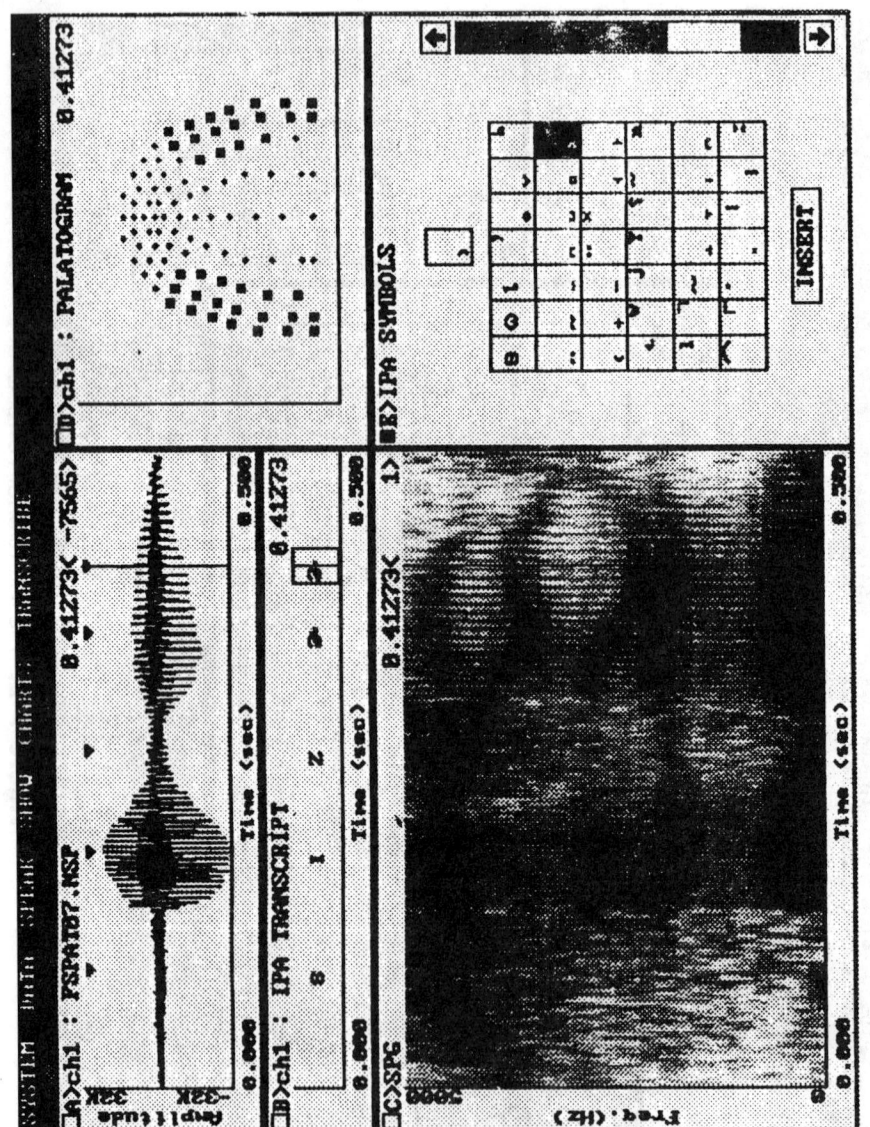

Figure 9–3. Sample of an analysis.

194

Integrating the extIPA Symbols

As we have noted in previous chapters, the 1989 Kiel Convention of the IPA recognized the need for symbols for the transcription of disordered speech. The result of the work of the Group on Disordered Speech and Voice Quality was the set of symbols now known as extIPA (Extensions to the IPA), and described in some detail in Chapter 4.

This set contains symbols and diacritics that cover a wide range of atypical segmental and suprasegmental articulations found in a variety of speech disorders. In addition, the VoQS symbols set (Ball, Esling, & Dickson, 1994, in press) contains means for marking a variety of voice qualities. Kay Elemetrics have funded a project to integrate the extIPA and VoQS symbols into the Phonetic Transcription Tutorial Program, and this work is currently underway, with an expected completion date in 1995.

Once this development is complete, a clinical tool will be available that will aid in the transcription of even the most atypical speech. The CSL Tutorial Program can be used with audio input alone, producing spectrographic traces, if required, or with EPG input alone, to produce palate contact diagrams. It is clearly, therefore, a flexible system and, as CSL can be used with other instrumentation, one can envisage future integration of information from electrolaryngography, endoscopic stroboscopy, and, perhaps, nasometry in the future.

Further still in the future of phonetic transcription lies the possibility of automated transcription systems. Speech recognition systems are developing rapidly, and one can certainly envisage equipment with which the normative data samples we have referred to could be compared automatically with input data and a match made with the nearest phonetic symbol. Considerable work will be needed to deal with disordered speech, however. Nevertheless, it is quite feasible that much, if not all, of the work involved in phonetic transcription may one day be computerized, and so relieving some of the time constraints on the busy speech-language clinician.

References

Abberton, E., & Fourcin, A. (1984). Electrolaryngography. In C. Code & M. J. Ball (Eds.), *Instrumentation in speech-language pathology* (pp. 62–78). San Diego: College-Hill Press.

Abberton, E., & Fourcin, A. (in press). Electrolaryngography. In C. Code & M. J. Ball (Eds.), *Instrumental clinical phonetics*. London: Whurr.

Abberton, E., Fourcin, A., Rosen, S., Walliker, J., Howard, D., Moore, B., Douek, E., & Frampton, S. (1985). Speech perceptual and productive rehabilitation in electrocochlear stimulation. In R. A. Schindler & M. M. Merzenich (Eds.), *Cochlear implants* (pp. 527–537). New York: Raven Press.

Abercrombie, D. (1964). *English phonetic texts*. London: Faber.

Abercrombie, D. (1967). *Elements of general phonetics*. Edinburgh: Edinburgh University Press.

Abercrombie, D. (1971). Some functions of silent stress. In J. Aitken, A. McIntosh, & H. Palsson (Eds.), *Edinburgh studies in English and Scots* (pp. 147-156). London: Longman.

Ainsworth, W. A., & Lindsay, D. (1984). Identification and discrimination of Halliday's primary tones. *Proceedings of the Institute of Acoustics, 6,* 379–383.

Ainsworth, W. A., & Lindsay, D. (1986). Perception of pitch movement on tonic syllables in British English. *Journal of the Acoustical Society of America, 79,* 472–480.

Allen, W. S. (1954). *Living English speech*. London: Longmans.

Altenberg, B. (1987). *Prosodic patterns in spoken English: Studies in the correspondence between prosody and grammar for text conversion.* (Lund Studies in English, 76.) Lund: Lund University Press.

Ansel, B., & Jucker, A. H. (1992). Learning linguistics with computers: HyperText as a key to linguistic networks. *Literary and Linguistic Computing, 7,* 124–131.

Anthony, J., & Hewlett, N. (1984). Aerometry. In C. Code & M. J. Ball (Eds.), *Instrumentation in speech-language pathology* (pp. 79–106) San Diego: College-Hill Press.

Armstrong, E. M. (1991). The potential of cohesion analysis in the analysis and treatment of aphasic discourse. *Clinical Linguistics and Phonetics, 5,* 39–51.

Armstrong, L. E., & Ward, I. C. (1926). *A handbook of English intonation.* Cambridge: Heffer.

Atkinson, J. M., & Heritage J. C. (Eds.). (1984). *Structures of social action: Studies in conversation analysis.* Cambridge: Cambridge University Press.

Bailey, C. J. N. (1978). Suggestions for improving the transcription of English segments. *Journal of Phonetics, 6,* 141–149.

Bailey, C. J. N. (1985). *English phonetic transcription.* Dallas: Summer Institute of Linguistics and University of Texas.

Ball, M. J. (1988). The contribution of speech pathology to the development of phonetic description. In M. J. Ball (Ed.), *Theoretical linguistics and disordered language* (pp. 168–188). San Diego: College-Hill Press.

Ball, M. J. (1992). Is a clinical sociolinguistics possible? *Clinical Linguistics and Phonetics, 6,* 155-160.

Ball, M. J. (1993). *Phonetics for speech pathology* (2nd ed.). London: Whurr.

Ball, M. J., & Code, C. (Eds.). (in press). *Instrumental clinical phonetics.* London: Whurr.

Ball, M. J., Code, C., Rahilly, J., & Hazlett, D. (1994). Non-segmental aspects of disordered speech: Developments in transcription. *Clinical Linguistics and Phonetics, 8,* 67–83.

Ball, M., Esling, J., & Dickson, C. (1994). *VoQS: Voice quality symbols.* Paper presented at the 4th International Clinical Phonetics and Linguistics Association Symposium, New Orleans.

Ball, M. J., Esling, J., & Dickson, C. (in press). The VoQS system for the transcription of voice quality. *Journal of the International Phonetic Association.*

Ball, M. J., & Gröne, B. (in press). Imaging techniques. In C. Code & M. J. Ball (Eds.), *Instrumental clinical phonetics.* London: Whurr.

Bell, A. M. (1867). *Visible speech.* London: Simpkin, Marshall & Co.

Bernhardt, B., & Ball, M. J. (1993). Characteristics of atypical speech currently not included in the Extensions to the IPA. *Journal of the International Phonetic Association, 23,* 35–38.

Bloch, B., & Trager, G. L. (1942). *Outline of linguistic analysis.* Baltimore: Linguistic Society of America.

Bloomfield, L. (1933). *Language.* New York: Holt, Rinehart and Winston.

Blumstein, S. E. (1991). The relation between phonetics and phonology. *Phonetica, 48,* 108–119.

Boas, F. (1911). *Handbook of American Indian languages* (Part I). Smithsonian Institution Bureau of American Ethnology, Bulletin 40. Washington, DC: U.S. Government Printing Office.

Boas, F., Goddard, P. E., Sapir, E., & Kroeber, A. L. (1916). *Phonetic transcription of American Indian languages: Report of Committee of American Anthropological Association.* Smithsonian Institution (Publication 2415, September). Also in Smithsonian Miscellaneous Collections 66 (1917), publication no. 2478, item no. 6. Washington DC: Smithsonian Institution.

Bolinger, D. (1964). *Intonation and its parts.* London: Edward Arnold.

Bolinger, D. (1989). *Intonation and its uses.* London: Edward Arnold.

Bowen, M., & Marks, J. (1992). *The pronunciation book.* London: Longman.

Brazil, D. C. (1975). *Discourse intonation.* Birmingham: English Language Research, University of Birmingham.

Brazil, D. C. (1978). *Discourse intonation II.* Birmingham: English Language Research, University of Birmingham.

Brazil, D. C. (1987). Representing pronunciation. In J. M. Sinclair (Ed.). *Looking up: An account of the COBUILD project in lexical computing* (pp. 160–166). London: Collins.

Brazil, D. C., Coulthard, M., & Johns, C. (1980). *Discourse intonation and language teaching.* London: Longman.

Brewster, K. (1989). Assessment of Prosody. In K. Grundy (Ed.), *Linguistics in clinical practice* (pp. 168–185). London: Taylor and Francis.

Brown, G. (1990). *Listening to spoken English* (2nd ed.). London: Longman.

Brown, G., Currie, K. L., & Kenworthy, J. (1980). *Questions of intonation.* London: Croom Helm.

Buckingham, H. W., & Yule, G. (1987). Phonemic false evaluation: Theoretical and clinical aspects. *Clinical Linguistics and Phonetics, 1,* 113–125.

Carney, E. (1979). Inappropriate abstraction in speech assessment procedures. *British Journal of Disorders of Communication, 14,* 123–35.

Carr, P. (1993). *Phonology.* London: Macmillan.

Catford, J. C. (1977). *Fundamental problems in phonetics.* Edinburgh: Edinburgh University Press.

Catford, J. C. (1988). *A Practical introduction to phonetics.* Oxford: Clarendon Press.

Chao, Y. R. & Yang, L. S. (1947). *Concise dictionary of spoken Chinese.* Cambridge, MA.: Harvard University Press.

Cheepen, C., & Monaghan, J. (1990). *Spoken English: A practical guide.* London: Pinter.

Chomsky, N., & Halle, M. (1968). *The sound pattern of English.* New York: Harper and Row.

Clark, J., & Yallop, C. (1990). *An introduction to phonetics and phonology.* Oxford: Blackwell.

Clark, J., & Yallop, C. (1995). *An introduction to phonetics and phonology* (2nd ed.). Oxford: Blackwell.

COBUILD Dictionary (Collins Birmingham University International Language Database). (1987). London: Collins.

Code, C., & Ball, M. J. (Eds.). (1984). *Instrumentation in speech-language pathology.* San Diego: College-Hill Press.

Code, C., & Ball, M. J. (1988). Apraxia of speech: the case for a cognitive phonetics. In M. J. Ball (Ed.), *Theoretical Linguistics and Disordered Language* (pp. 152–167). San Diego: College-Hill Press.

Cowie, R. I. D., & Douglas-Cowie, E. (1983). Speech production in profound postlingual deafness. In M. E. Lutman, & M. P. Haggard (Eds.), *Hearing science and hearing disorders* (pp. 183-230). London: Academic Press.

Cruttenden, A. (1986). *Intonation.* Cambridge: Cambridge University Press.

Crystal, D. (1969). *Prosodic systems and intonation in English.* Cambridge: Cambridge University Press.

Crystal, D. (1984). *Linguistic encounters with language handicap*. Oxford: Blackwell.

Crystal, D. (1985). Things to remember when transcribing speech. *Journal of Child Language Teaching and Therapy, 2*, 235–239.

Crystal, D., & Davy, D. (1969). *Investigating English style*. London: Longman.

Crystal, D., & Davy, D. (1975). *Advanced English conversation*. London: Longman.

Crystal, D., & Quirk, R. (1964). *Systems of prosodic and paralinguistic features in English*. The Hague: Mouton.

Cutler, A. (1980). Errors of stress and intonation. In V. Fromkin (Ed.), *Errors in linguistic performance—Slips of the tongue, ear, pen and hand* (pp. 67-80). London: Academic Press.

Dalton, P., & Hardcastle, W. J. (1977). *Disorders of fluency*. London: Edward Arnold.

Diehl, R. L. (1991). The role of phonetics within the study of language. *Phonetica, 48*, 120–134.

Douglas-Cowie, E., & Cowie, R. (1989). Speech disorder as a sociolinguistic problem. *York Papers in Linguistics, 13*, 155–166.

Duckworth, M., Allen, G. Hardcastle, W. J., & Ball, M. J. (1990). Extensions to the International Phonetic Alphabet for the transcription of atypical speech. *Clinical Linguistics and Phonetics, 4*, 273–280.

Edwards, M. L. (1986). *Introduction to applied phonetics: Laboratory workbook*. San Diego: College-Hill Press.

Edwards, S., & Garman, M. (1989). Case study of a fluent aphasic. In P. Grunwell & A. James (Eds.), *The functional evaluation of language disorders* (pp. 163–181). London: Croom Helm.

Evershed-Martin, S. (1989). Assessment of Speech Production. In K. Grundy (Ed.), *Linguistics in clinical practice* (pp. 50-70). London: Taylor and Francis.

Farmer, A. (1984). Spectrography. In C. Code & M. J. Ball (Eds.), *Instrumentation in speech-language pathology* (pp. 21-40). San Diego: College-Hill Press.

Farmer, A. (in press). Spectrography. In C. Code & M. J. Ball (Eds.), *Instrumental clinical phonetics*. London: Whurr.

Fawcett, R., & Perkins, M. (1980). *Child language transcripts 6–12*. Pontypridd: Polytechnic of Wales. [now University of Glamorgan]

Francis, G., & Hunston, S. (1992). Analyzing everyday conversation. In M. Coulthard (Ed.), *Advances in spoken discourse analysis* (pp. 123-161). London: Routledge.

Gandour, J. (1978). The perception of tone. In Fromkin, V. (Ed.), *Tone: A linguistic survey* (pp. 41–76). New York: Academic Press.

Gimson, A. C. (1989). *An introduction to the pronunciation of English* (4th ed.). London: Edward Arnold.

Gleason, H. A. (1955). *Workbook in descriptive linguistics*. New York: Holt Rinehart and Winston.

Grice, P. (1975). Logic and conversation. In P. Cole & J. Morgan (Eds.), *Syntax and semantics 3: Speech acts* (pp. 41–58). London: Academic Press.

Grunwell, P. (1985). Comment on the terms 'phonetics' and 'phonology' as applied in the investigation of speech disorders. *British Journal of Disorders of Communication, 20*, 165–170.

Grunwell, P. (1987). *Clinical phonology* (2nd. ed). London: Croom Helm.

Grunwell, P., & Russell, J. (1988). Phonological development in children with cleft lip and palate. *Clinical Linguistics and Phonetics, 2,* 75–95.

Gussenhoven, C. (1984). *On the grammar and semantics of sentence accents.* Dordrecht: Foris.

Halliday, M. A. K. (1967). *Intonation and grammar in British English.* The Hague: Mouton.

Halliday, M. A. K. (1970). *A course in spoken English: Intonation.* Oxford: Oxford University Press.

Halliday, M. A. K. (1994). *An introduction to functional grammar* (2nd ed.). London: Edward Arnold.

Hardcastle, W. J., & Gibbon, F. (in press). Electropalatography. In C. Code & M. J. Ball (Eds.), *Instrumental clinical phonetics.* London: Whurr.

Hardcastle, W. J., Jones, W., Knight, C., Trudgeon, A., & Calder, G. (1989). New developments in electropalatography: A state-of-the-art report. *Clinical Linguistics and Phonetics, 3,* 1–38.

Harris, J., & Cottam, P. (1985). Phonetic features and phonological features in speech assessment. *British Journal of Disorders of Communication, 20,* 61–74.

Hawkins, P. (1985). A tutorial comment on Harris and Cottam. *British Journal of Disorders of Communication, 20,* 75–80.

Hawkins, P. (1989). Discourse aphasia. In P. Grunwell & A. James (Eds.). *The functional evaluation of language disorders* (pp. 183–199). London: Croom Helm.

Henderson, E. J. A. (1949). Prosodies in Siamese. *Asia Major (New Series), 1,* 189–215.

Hewlett, N. (1985). Phonological versus phonetic disorders: some suggested modifications to the current use of the distinction. *British Journal of Disorders of Communication, 20,* 155–164.

Hockett, C. F. (1955). *A manual of phonology.* Baltimore: Waverley Press. Also, IJAL Memoir II. *International Journal of American Linguistics, 21,* (4), part I. Chicago: University of Chicago Press.

Hodson, B. W. (1980). *The assessment of phonological processes.* Danville, IL: Interstate Inc.

Holmes, J. (1992). *An introduction to sociolinguistics.* London: Longman.

Howard, S. (1993). Articulatory constraints on a phonological system: a case study of cleft palate speech. *Clinical Linguistics and Phonetics, 7,* 299–317.

Ingram, D. (1976). *Phonological disability in children.* London: Edward Arnold.

Ingram, D. (1981). *Procedures for the phonological analysis of children's language.* Baltimore: University Park Press.

International African Institute. (1930). *Practical orthography of African languages.* London: IAI.

International Phonetic Association. (1949). *The Principles of the International Phonetic Association.* London: Department of Phonetics, University College (reprinted 1978: Dept. of Phonetics and Linguistics, University College London).

International Phonetic Association. (1989). Report on the 1989 Kiel Convention. *Journal of the International Phonetic Association, 19,* 67–80.

International Phonetic Association. (1993). Council actions on revisions of the IPA. *Journal of the International Phonetic Association, 23,* 32–34.

Jannedy, S., Poletto, R., & Weldon, T. (1994). *Language files.* Ohio State University, Department of Linguistics.

Jassem, W., Hill, D. R., & Witten, I. H. (1984). Isochrony in English speech. In D. Gibbon & H. Richter (Eds.), *Intonation, accent and rhythm* (pp. 203–225). Berlin: de Gruyter.

Jefferson, G. (1988). Preliminary notes on a possible metric which provides for a standard maximum silence of approximately one second in conversation. In D. Roger & P. Bull (Eds.), *Conversation* (pp. 166-196). Clevedon: Multilingual Matters.

JIPA: Journal of the International Phonetic Association (formerly *Le Maître Phonétique*). London: International Phonetic Association.

Johnson, S. (1755). *Dictionary of the English language.* London: Robert Dodsley.

Jones, D. (1918). *An outline of English phonetics.* Cambridge: Heffer.

Jones, D. (1960). *An outline of English phonetics* (9th ed.). Cambridge: Heffer.

Kearns, K. P., & Simmons, N. N. (1988). Interobserver reliability and perceptual ratings: more than meets the ear. *Journal of Speech and Hearing Research, 30,* 131–136.

Kenyon, J. S. (1950). *American pronunciation.* (10th ed.). Ann Arbor, MI: George Wahr.

Kingdon, R. (1958). *The groundwork of English intonation.* London: Longman.

Klee, T., & Ingrisano, D. (1992). *Clarifying the transcription of indeterminable utterances.* Paper presented at ASHA Convention, San Antonio.

Knowles, G. (1986). The automatic accentuation of English texts. *Lancaster Papers in Linguistics, 42.*

Knowles, G. (1987). *Patterns of spoken English.* London: Longman

Kramer, E. (1963). Judgement of personality characteristics and emotions form nonverbal properties of speech. *Psychological Bulletin, 60,* 408–420.

Kreidler, C.W. (1989). *The pronunciation of English: A course book in phonology.* Oxford: Blackwell.

Ladefoged, P. (1968). *A phonetic Study of West African Languages.* Cambridge: Cambridge University Press.

Ladefoged, P. (1975). *A course in phonetics.* New York: Harcourt, Brace Jovanovich.

Ladefoged, P. (1982). *A course in phonetics* (2nd ed.). New York: Harcourt, Brace Jovanovich.

Lass, R. (1984). *Phonology: an introduction to basic concepts.* Cambridge: Cambridge University Press.

Laufer, A. (1991). The glottal fricatives. *Journal of the International Phonetic Association, 21,* 91–93.

Laver, J. (1980). *The phonetic description of voice quality.* Cambridge: Cambridge University Press.

Laver, J. (1994). *Principles of Phonetics.* Cambridge: Cambridge University Press.

Leben, W. R. (1980). *Suprasegmental phonology.* New York: Garland.

Leder, S., Spitzer, J., Milner, P., Flevaris-Phillips, C., Kirchner, C., & Richardson, F. (1987). Speaking rate of adventitiously deaf male cochlear implant candidates. *Journal of the Acoustical Society of America, 82,* 843–846.

Leff, J., & Abberton, E. (1981). Voice pitch measurements in schizophrenia and depression. *Psychological Medicine, 11,* 849–852.

Lehiste, I. (1980). *Phonetic characteristics of discourse.* Tokyo: Acoustical Society of Japan.

Lehiste, I. (1982). Some phonetic characteristics of discourse. *Studia Linguistica, 36,* 117–130.

Lenneberg, E. H. (1967). *Biological foundations of language.* New York: John Wiley.

Lesser, R., & Milroy, L. (1993). *Linguistics and aphasia*. London: Longman.

Lewis, J. R. (1972). *A concise pronouncing dictionary of British and American English*. Oxford: OUP.

Liberman, M. (1979). *The intonational system of English*. New York: Garland.

Longman Pronunciation Dictionary. (1990). London: Longman.

MacCarthy, P. (1952). *English pronunciation* (4th ed.). Cambridge: Heffer.

MacCarthy, P. (1978). *The teaching of pronunciation*. Cambridge: Cambridge University Press.

MacMahon, M. K. C. (1986). The International Phonetic Association: The first 100 years. *Journal of the International Phonetic Association, 16*, 30–38.

Malmberg, B. (Ed.) (1968). *Manual of phonetics*. Amsterdam: North Holland.

Miller, J. & Tench, P. (1982). Aspects of Hausa intonation, II. *Journal of the International Phonetic Association, 12*, 78–93.

Nilsonne, A., Sundberg, J., Ternstrom, S., & Askenfelt, A. (1988). Measuring the rate of change of voice fundamental frequency in fluent speech during mental depression. *Journal of the Acoustical Society of America, 83*, 716–728.

O'Connor, J. D. (1973). *Phonetics*. Harmondsworth: Penguin.

O'Connor, J. D. (1980). *Better English pronunciation* (2nd ed.). Cambridge: Cambridge University Press.

O'Connor, J. D., & Arnold, G. E. (1961). *Intonation of colloquial English*. London: Longman.

O'Connor, J. D., & Arnold, G. E. (1973). *Intonation of colloquial English* (2nd ed.). London: Longman.

Olive, J. P. (1975). Fundamental frequency rules for the synthesis of simple declarative English sentences. *Journal of the Acoustical Society of America, 57*, 476–482.

The Oxford English dictionary. (1933). Oxford: Oxford University Press.

Oxford advanced learners dictionary. (4th ed.). (1989). Edited by A. P. Cowie, Oxford: Oxford University Press.

The Oxford senior dictionary. (1982). Oxford: Oxford University Press.

Palmer, H. E. (1922). *English intonation (with systematic exercises)*. Cambridge: Heffer.

Parker, A. (1983). Speech conservation. *British Journal of Audiology, 18*, 39–45

Pike, E. V. (1963). *Dictation exercises in phonetics*. Santa Ana CA: Summer Institute of Linguistics.

Pike, K. L. (1943). *Phonetics*. Ann Arbor MI: University of Michigan Press.

Pike, K. L. (1945). *The intonation of American English*. Ann Arbor MI: University of Michigan Press.

Pike, K. L. (1947). *Phonemics: A technique for reducing languages to writing*. Ann Arbor MI: University of Michigan Press.

Pike, K. L. (1948). *Tone languages*. Ann Arbor MI: University of Michigan Press.

Pike, K. L. (1962). Practical phonetics of rhythm waves. *Phonetica, 8*, 9–30.

Potter, J., & Wetherell, M. (1987). *Discourse and social psychology*. London: Sage.

PRDS (1980). Progress report. *British Journal of Disorders of Communication, 15*, 215–220.

PRDS (1983). The phonetic representation of disordered speech. *King's Fund Project Paper, 38*. London: The King's Fund.

Pullum, G. K., & Ladusaw, W. A. (1986). *Phonetic symbol guide*. Chicago: University of Chicago Press.

Quirk, R., Duckworth, A. P., Svartvik, J., Rusiecki, J. P. L., & Colin, A. J. T. (1964). Studies in the correspondence of prosodic to grammatical features in English. In *Proceedings of the 9th International Congress of Linguists*. The Hague: Mouton, 679–691.

Rahilly, J. (1991). *Intonation Patterns in Normal-hearing and Postlingually-deafened Adults in Belfast*. Unpublished doctoral dissertation, Queen's University, Belfast.

Roach, P. (1991). *English phonetics and phonology: A practical course* (2nd. ed). Cambridge: Cambridge University Press.

Rogers, H. (1991). *Theoretical and practical phonetics*. Toronto: Copp Clark Pittman.

Rosen, S. M., Fourcin, A. J., & Moore, B. C. J. (1981) Voice pitch as an aid to lipreading. *Nature, 5811*, 150–152 .

Rosenthal, J. B. (1989). A computer-assisted phonetic transcription skill development program. *Folia Phoniatrica, 41,* 243.

Ryalls, J., Bédard, F., Chamberland, J., & Larouche, A. (1993). Phonemic substitutions of French-speaking children with profound hearing impairment. *Clinical Linguistics and Phonetics, 7,* 113–118.

Sag, I., & Liberman, M. (1975) The intonational disambiguation of indirect speech acts. *Papers from the 11th Regional Meeting, Chicago Linguistic Society*, 487–497.

Samar, V. J., & Metz, D. E. (1991). Scaling and transcription measures of intelligibility for populations with disordered speech—where's the beef? *Journal of Speech and Hearing Research, 34,* 699–702.

Sapir, E. (1925). Sound patterns in language. *Language, 1,* 37–51.

Shriberg, L., & Kent, R. D. (1982). *Clinical phonetics*. New York: Macmillan.

Shriberg, L., & Kwiatowski, J. (1980). *Natural process analysis (NPA): A procedure for phonological analysis of continuous speech samples*. New York: Macmillan.

Shriberg, L., Hincke, R., & Trost-Steffen, C. (1987). A procedure to select and train persons for narrow phonetic transcription by consensus. *Clinical Linguistics and Phonetics, 1,* 171–189.

Shriberg, L., & Lof, G. (1991). Reliability studies in broad and narrow transcription. *Clinical Linguistics and Phonetics, 5,* 225–279.

Siren, K. A., & Wilcox, K. A. (1990). The utility of phonetic versus orthographic transcription methods. *Journal of Child Language Teaching and Therapy, 6,* 127–146.

Slembrouck, S. (1992). The parliamentary Hansard verbatim report: the written construction of spoken discourse. *Language and Literature, 1,* 101–119.

Smalley, W. A. (1963). *Manual of articulatory phonetics* (rev. ed.). Tarrytown, NY: Practical Anthropology.

Smith, C. R. (1975). *Residual hearing and speech production in deaf children*. New York: Rinehart and Winston.

Stackhouse, J., & Snowling, M. (1992). Developmental verbal dyspraxia II: A developmental perspective on two case studies. *European Journal of Disorders of Communication, 27,* 35–54.

Strevens, P. (1978). A rationale for teaching pronunciation. *English Language Teaching Journal, 28,* 182–189.

Svartvik, J., & Quirk, R. (1980). *A corpus of English conversation*. Lund: Gleerup.

Sweet, H. (1877). *A handbook of phonetics* (Republished 1970). College Park, MD: McGrath.

Sweet, H. (1880-1881). Sound notation. *Transactions of the Philological Society*, 177–235. (reprinted in E. J. A. Henderson (Ed.), *The indispensable foundation*, London: Oxford University Press. 1971.)

Tatham, M. A. A. (1984). Towards a *cognitive* phonetics. *Journal of Phonetics, 12*, 37–47.

Tench, P. (1988). The stylistic potential of intonation. In N. Coupland (Ed.), *Styles of discourse* (pp. 50–84). London: Croom Helm.

Tench, P. (1990). *The roles of intonation in English discourse*. Frankfurt a M: Peter Lang.

The sounds of the International Phonetic Alphabet (free to IPA members). IPA, Linguistics Department, UCLA, Los Angeles *or* IPA, Linguistics Department, University of Leeds, UK.

Tingsabadh, M. R. K., & Abramson, A. S. (1993). Thai. *Journal of the International Phonetic Association, 23*, 24–28.

Trager, G. L. (1964). *Phonetics: glossary and tables*. (2nd ed., rev.). *(Studies in Linguistics: Occasional Papers* 6.). Buffalo, NY: George L. Trager.

Trager, G. L., & Smith, H. L., Jr. (1951). *An outline of English structure. (Studies in Linguistics: Occasional Papers* 3). Norman, OK: Battenburg Press.

Trudgill, P. (1983). *Sociolinguistics*. London: Longman.

Vieregge, W. (1987). Basic aspects of phonetic segmental transcription. *Zeitschrift für Dialektologie und Linguistik.Beihefte, 54*, 5–55.

Ward, I. C. (1945). *The phonetics of English* (4th ed.). Cambridge: Heffer.

Waters, T. (1986). Speech therapy with cochlear implant wearers. *British Journal of Audiology, 20*, 35–43.

Webster, N. (1828). *An American dictionary of the English language.* Springfield, MA: Merriam.

Websters third new international dictionary of the English language. (1961). Springfield, MA: Merriam.

Weiner, F. F. (1979). *Phonological process analysis (PPA).* Baltimore: University Park Press.

Wells, J. C., & Colson, G. (1973). *Practical phonetics*. London: Pitman.

Wells, W. (1992). *Phonetic aspects of focus in London Jamaican.* Paper presented at the BAAP Colloquium, Cambridge.

Wells, W. (1994). Junction in developmental speech disorders: A case study. *Clinical Linguistics and Phonetics, 8*, 1–25.

Westermann, D., & Ward, I. C. (1933). *Practical phonetics for students of African languages.* (Republished 1990. Edited by J. Kelly. London: Kegan Paul International).

Yule, G. (1980). Speakers topics and major paratones. *Lingua, 52*, 33–47.

Zajac, D., & Yates, C. (in press) Speech aerodynamics. In C. Code & M. J. Ball (Eds.), *Instrumental clinical phonetics.* London: Whurr.

Appendix

THE INTERNATIONAL PHONETIC ALPHABET (revised to 1993)

CONSONANTS (PULMONIC)

	Bilabial	Labiodental	Dental	Alveolar	Postalveolar	Retroflex	Palatal	Velar	Uvular	Pharyngeal	Glottal
Plosive	p b			t d		ʈ ɖ	c ɟ	k g	q ɢ		ʔ
Nasal	m	ɱ		n		ɳ	ɲ	ŋ	N		
Trill	ʙ			r					R		
Tap or Flap				ɾ		ɽ					
Fricative	ɸ β	f v	θ ð	s z	ʃ ʒ	ʂ ʐ	ç ʝ	x ɣ	χ ʁ	ħ ʕ	h ɦ
Lateral fricative				ɬ ɮ							
Approximant		ʋ		ɹ		ɻ	j	ɰ			
Lateral approximant				l		ɭ	ʎ	L			

Where symbols appear in pairs, the one to the right represents a voiced consonant. Shaded areas denote articulations judged impossible.

CONSONANTS (NON-PULMONIC)

Clicks	Voiced implosives	Ejectives
ʘ Bilabial	ɓ Bilabial	ʼ as in:
ǀ Dental	ɗ Dental/alveolar	pʼ Bilabial
ǃ (Post)alveolar	ʄ Palatal	tʼ Dental/alveolar
ǂ Palatoalveolar	ɠ Velar	kʼ Velar
ǁ Alveolar lateral	ʛ Uvular	sʼ Alveolar fricative

VOWELS

```
          Front        Central        Back
Close     i • y ——— ɨ • ʉ ——— ɯ • u
             ɪ  ʏ              ʊ
Close-mid  e • ø ——— ɘ • ɵ ——— ɤ • o
                         ə
Open-mid     ɛ • œ — ɜ • ɞ — ʌ • ɔ
                æ         ɐ
Open           a • ɶ ——— ɑ • ɒ
```

Where symbols appear in pairs, the one to the right represents a rounded vowel.

OTHER SYMBOLS

ʍ Voiceless labial-velar fricative
w Voiced labial-velar approximant
ɥ Voiced labial-palatal approximant
ʜ Voiceless epiglottal fricative
ʢ Voiced epiglottal fricative
ʡ Epiglottal plosive

ɕ ʑ Alveolo-palatal fricatives
ɺ Alveolar lateral flap
ɧ Simultaneous ʃ and X

Affricates and double articulations can be represented by two symbols joined by a tie bar if necessary.

k͡p t͡s

SUPRASEGMENTALS

ˈ	Primary stress	ˌfoʊnəˈtɪʃən
ˌ	Secondary stress	
ː	Long	eː
ˑ	Half-long	eˑ
˘	Extra-short	ĕ
.	Syllable break	ɹi.ækt
|	Minor (foot) group	
‖	Major (intonation) group	
‿	Linking (absence of a break)	

TONES & WORD ACCENTS

LEVEL		CONTOUR	
e̋ or ˥	Extra high	ě or ˩	Rising
é ˦	High	ê ˥	Falling
ē ˧	Mid	e᷄ ˦	High rising
è ˨	Low	e᷅ ˩	Low rising
ȅ ˩	Extra low	e᷈ ˧	Rising-falling
↓ Downstep		↗ Global rise	etc.
↑ Upstep		↘ Global fall	

DIACRITICS

Diacritics may be placed above a symbol with a descender, e.g. ŋ̊

̥	Voiceless	n̥ d̥	̤	Breathy voiced	b̤ a̤	̪	Dental	t̪ d̪
̬	Voiced	s̬ t̬	̰	Creaky voiced	b̰ a̰	̺	Apical	t̺ d̺
ʰ	Aspirated	tʰ dʰ	̼	Linguolabial	t̼ d̼	̻	Laminal	t̻ d̻
̹	More rounded	ɔ̹	ʷ	Labialized	tʷ dʷ	̃	Nasalized	ẽ
̜	Less rounded	ɔ̜	ʲ	Palatalized	tʲ dʲ	ⁿ	Nasal release	dⁿ
̟	Advanced	u̟	ˠ	Velarized	tˠ dˠ	ˡ	Lateral release	dˡ
̠	Retracted	i̠	ˤ	Pharyngealized	tˤ dˤ	̚	No audible release	d̚
̈	Centralized	ë	̴	Velarized or pharyngealized	ɫ			
̽	Mid-centralized	e̽	̝	Raised	e̝ (ɹ̝ = voiced alveolar fricative)			
̩	Syllabic	ɹ̩	̞	Lowered	e̞ (β̞ = voiced bilabial approximant)			
̯	Non-syllabic	e̯	̘	Advanced Tongue Root	e̘			
˞	Rhoticity	ɚ	̙	Retracted Tongue Root	e̙			

IPA Chart 1993. (Reprinted with permission.)

extIPA SYMBOLS FOR DISORDERED SPEECH
(Revised to 1994)

CONSONANTS (other than those on the IPA Chart)

	bilabial	labiodental	dentolabial	labioalv.	linguolabial	interdental	bidental	alveolar	velar	velophar.
Plosive	p̪ b̪		p̪͆ ɓ̪	p̪ b̪	t̼ d̼	t̪͆ d̪͆				
Nasal			m̪͆	m̪	n̼	n̪͆				
Trill					r̼	r̪͆				
Fricative median			f̪͆ v̪͆	f̪ v̪	θ̼ ð̼	θ̪͆ ð̪͆	ɦ̪͆ ɦ̪͆			fŋ
Fricative lateral+median								ʪ ʫ		
Fricative nareal	m̊ ͋							n̊ ͋	ŋ̊ ͋	
Percussive	w̜ w̜						ʭ			
Approximant lateral					l̼	l̪͆				

DIACRITICS

↔	labial spreading	s̪	͈	strong articulation	f͈	˷	denasal	m̃̃
˞	dentolabial	v̂	˷	weak articulation	v̬	˙̃	nasal escape	ṽ̃
˷	interdental/bidental	n̪͆	\	reiterated articulation	p\p\p	ꜝ	velopharyngeal friction	s̃
=	alveolar	l̪	↟	whistled articulation	s̝	↓	ingressive airflow	p↓
˷	linguolabial	d̼	→	sliding articulation	θs	↑	egressive airflow	!↑

CONNECTED SPEECH

(.)	short pause
(..)	medium pause
(...)	long pause
ʃ	loud speech [{ʃ laʊd ʃ}]
ʃʃ	louder speech [{ʃʃ laʊdə ʃʃ}]
p	quiet speech [{p kwaɪət p}]
pp	quieter speech [{pp kwaɪətə pp}]
allegro	fast speech [{allegro fɑːst allegro}]
lento	slow speech [{ lento sloʊ lento}]
crescendo, ralentando, etc may also be used

VOICING

	pre-voicing	ˌz
	post-voicing	zˌ
₍ₐ₎	partial devoicing	₍z₎
₍ₐ	initial partial devoicing	₍z
ₐ₎	final partial devoicing	z₎
₍ᵥ₎	partial voicing	₍s₎
₍ᵥ	initial partial voicing	₍s
ᵥ₎	final partial voicing	s₎
=	unaspirated	p=
ʰ	pre-aspiration	ʰp

OTHERS

(⎻)	indeterminate sound	( )	silent articulation	(ʃ)
(V̄)	indeterminate vowel	(( ))	extraneous noise	((2 sylls))
(Pl)	indeterminate plosive	*	sound with no symbol available	
(Pl,vls)	indeterminate voiceless plosive, etc		(to be described elsewhere)	

ExtIPA Chart 1994. (Reprinted with permission.)

VoQS: Voice Quality Symbols

AIRSTREAM TYPES

Œ	oesophageal speech	Ɯ	electrolarynx speech
Ю	tracheo-oesophageal speech	↓	pulmonic ingressive speech

PHONATION TYPES

V	modal voice	F	falsetto
W	whisper	C	creak
V̰	whispery voice (murmur)	V̰	creaky voice
V̤	breathy voice	C̣	whispery creak
V!	harsh voice	V!!	ventricular phonation
V̰!!	diplophonia	V̰!!	whispery ventricular phon.
V̩	anterior or pressed phonation	W̲	posterior whisper

SUPRALARYNGEAL SETTINGS

L̬	raised larynx	L̬	lowered larynx
Vᶿ	labialized voice (open round)	Vʷ	labialized voice (close round)
V̴	spread-lip voice	Vᶹ	labio-dentalized voice
V̬	linguo-apicalized voice	V̥	linguo-laminalized voice
V˞	retroflex voice	V̪	dentalized voice
V̳	alveolarized voice	V̺ʲ	palatoalveolarized voice
Vʲ	palatalized voice	Vˠ	velarized voice
Vʁ	uvularized voice	Vˤ	pharyngealized voice
V̰ˤ	laryngo-pharyngealized voice	Vᴴ	faucalized voice
Ṽ	nasalized voice	V̟	denasalized voice
J̞	open jaw voice	J̝	close jaw voice
J̪	right offset jaw voice	J̺	left offset jaw voice
J̟	protruded jaw voice	Θ	protruded tongue voice

USE OF LABELED BRACES & NUMERALS TO MARK STRETCHES OF
SPEECH AND DEGREES AND COMBINATIONS OF VOICE QUALITY

['ðɪs ɪz 'nɔˑməl 'vɔɪs {3V! 'ðɪs ɪz 'veri 'hɑˑʃ 'vɔɪs 3V!} 'ðɪs ɪz 'nɔˑməl 'vɔɪs
wʌns 'mɔˑ {L̬1V! 'ðɪs ɪz 'les 'hɑˑʃ 'vɔɪs wɪð 'loʊəd 'læɹɪŋks 1V!L̬}]

VoQS Chart. (Reprinted with permission.)

Index